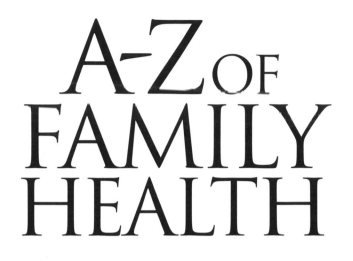

# A-Z OF FAMILY HEALTH

# LONDON, NEW YORK, MUNICH, MELBOURNE, DELHI

Produced for Dorling Kindersley by
The Brown Reference Group plc, 8 Chapel Place, Rivington Street, London, EC2A 3DQ

The information in this publication has previously been published in the *A-Z Family Medical Encyclopedia*, copyright © 1990, 1995, 1999, 2004 Dorling Kindersley Limited; *Home Doctor*, text copyright © 2004 Michael Peters; *Complete Family Health Guide*, copyright © 2000 Dorling Kindersley Limited; *Nutrition for Life*, text copyright © 2005 Lisa Hark and Darwin Deen; *Encyclopedia of Natural Healing*, text copyright © 1997 Anne Woodham and David Peters; and *Human Body* © 2001 Dorling Kindersley Limited

Published in 2005 by MDS BOOKS/MEDIASAT Group
in association with MediaFund Limited

MediaSat: C/ Agustín de Betancourt, 19, 28003 Madrid, Spain
www.mediasatgroup.com

MediaFund Limited: Rutland House, Rutland Gardens, London SW7 1BX
www.mediafund.co.uk

A CIP catalogue record for this publication is available from the British Library
ISBN: 84-9789-773-0 (The Collection)
ISBN: 84-9789-776-5 (Volume 3)
ISSN: 1745-2732

Not to be sold separately from the *Daily Mail*

Colour reproduction by Colourscan, Singapore
Printed and bound in the E.U.

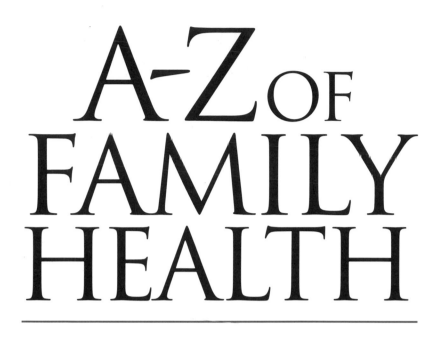

# A-Z OF FAMILY HEALTH

## Volume 3

Artifical kidney – Biofeedback

# Artificial kidney

The common name for the machine used in *dialysis*.

# Artificial limb

See *prosthesis*.

# Artificial respiration

See *rescue breathing*.

# Artificial saliva

A preparation used to relieve a persistently dry mouth, which may be a side effect of certain drugs or *radiotherapy* or may be due to *Sjögren's syndrome* (an autoimmune disorder in which the immune system attacks the body's own tissues). Artificial saliva, as a spray, gel, or pastilles, is formulated to resemble natural saliva as closely as possible.

# Artificial tears

Preparations that are used to supplement tear production in disorders, such as *keratoconjunctivitis sicca*, that cause dry eye and to relieve irritation.

# Art therapy

See box on page 134.

# Asbestosis

See *asbestos-related diseases*.

# Asbestos-related diseases

A variety of diseases that are caused by inhalation of asbestos fibres. Asbestos is a fibrous mineral formerly used as a heat- and fire-resistant insulating material. There are three main types: white, which is widely used, blue, and brown. Blue and brown are the most dangerous types. The use of all types is now carefully controlled.

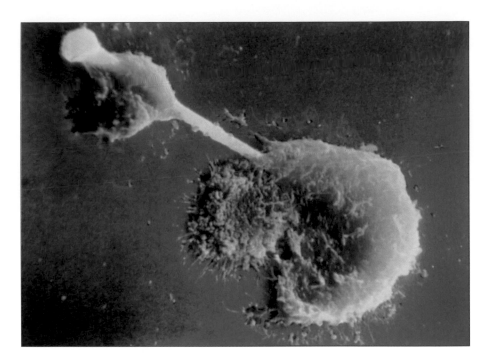

**An inhaled asbestos fibre** *in a lung (shown in an electron micrograph) impales and kills a macrophage (a scavenger cell that would normally engulf and destroy foreign particles in the lungs).*

### TYPES

In asbestosis, widespread fine scarring occurs in the lungs. The disease causes breathlessness and a dry cough, eventually leading to severe disability and death. Asbestosis develops mostly in industrial workers who have been heavily exposed to asbestos. The period from initial exposure to development of the disease is usually at least 20 years. Diagnosis is by *chest X-ray*. Asbestosis increases the risk of developing *lung cancer*.

*Mesothelioma* is a cancerous tumour of the *pleura* (the membrane surrounding the lungs) or the *peritoneum* (the membrane lining the abdominal cavity). In the pleura, mesotheliomas cause pain and breathlessness; in the peritoneum they cause enlargement of the abdomen and intestinal obstruction. The condition cannot be treated and usually leads to death within one or two years. The average interval between initial exposure to asbestos and death is between 20 and 30 years. Mesothelioma affects people who have been exposed to blue or brown asbestos.

Diffuse pleural thickening is a condition in which the outer and inner layers of the pleura become thickened, and excess fluid may accumulate in the cavity between them. This combination restricts the ability of the lungs to expand, resulting in shortness of breath. The condition may develop even after short exposure to asbestos.

# Ascariasis

Infestation with the roundworm *ASCARIS LUMBRICOIDES*, which lives in the small intestine of its human host. Ascariasis is common worldwide, especially in the tropics.

One or several worms may be present, but symptoms usually only occur with heavy infestation.

### CAUSES

The parasite that causes ascariasis is a pale, cylindrical, tapered roundworm, which reaches between 15 and 35 cm in length in its adult form.

Ascariasis is spread by ingestion of worm eggs, usually from food grown in soil that has been contaminated by human faeces. In some dry, windy climates, airborne eggs may be swallowed after being blown into the mouth.

## SYMPTOMS

Light infestation may cause no symptoms, although mild nausea, abdominal pain, and irregular bowel movements may occur. A worm may be passed via the rectum, or it may be vomited. A large number of worms may compete with the host for food, leading to malnutrition and *anaemia*, which, in children, can retard growth.

## TREATMENT

The worm infestation is treated with *anthelmintic drugs*, such as levamisole, which usually bring about complete recovery. The worms are passed out of the body via the rectum some days after the drug is taken.

# Ascites

Excess fluid in the peritoneal cavity, the space between the two layers of the peritoneum (the membranes that line the inside of the abdominal wall and cover the abdominal organs).

## CAUSES

Ascites may occur in any condition that causes generalized *oedema* (excessive accumulation of fluid in the body tissues), such as in congestive *heart failure*, *nephrotic syndrome*, and *cirrhosis* of the liver.

Ascites may occur in *cancer* if metastases (secondary growths) from a cancer elsewhere in the body develop in the peritoneum. The condition also occurs if *tuberculosis* affects the abdomen.

## SYMPTOMS

Ascites causes abdominal swelling and discomfort. Additionally, it may cause breathing difficulty as a result of pressure on, and the immobilization of, the diaphragm, the sheet of muscle that separates the thorax (the chest) from the abdomen.

## DIAGNOSIS

The doctor diagnoses the cause of ascites by analysing a sample of ascitic fluid taken via a sterile needle inserted through the abdominal wall.

## TREATMENT

The underlying cause is treated if possible. *Diuretic drugs*, particularly *spironolactone*, are often used to treat ascites associated with cirrhosis. If the ascites is causing discomfort or breathing difficulty, fluid can be drained from the peritoneal cavity.

# Ascorbic acid

The chemical name for *vitamin C*.

# ASD

The abbreviation for *atrial septal defect*.

# Aseptic necrosis

Death of an area of bone tissue in the absence of infection. The cause of aseptic necrosis is almost always damage to the blood supply to bone, often as a result of a fracture.

In some cases, the condition is associated with treatment with *corticosteroid drugs*.

Aseptic necrosis often results in chronic (long-term) pain and may cause stiffness in adjacent joints.

Early treatment of fractures reduces the risk of the condition developing.

The head of the *femur* (thigh-bone) and the *scaphoid* (a bone in the wrist) are particularly likely to be affected by aseptic necrosis.

Aseptic necrosis may be diagnosed from *X-rays*; the area of bone that is affected appears denser than the surrounding bone.

---

## LIFE CYCLE OF THE ASCARIS WORM

People usually become infested with roundworms such as *ASCARIS LUMBRICOIDES* by eating food or drinking water contaminated with the worm eggs. Once swallowed, the worm eggs hatch into larvae in the intestine. The larvae then travel in the blood to the lungs and later return to the intestine, where they develop into adults, breed, and lay eggs.

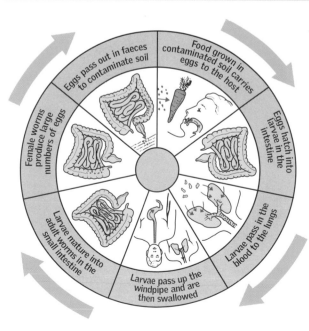

**Parasitic cycle**
*The person becomes infested by swallowing the eggs, which may be in contaminated water or on food grown in contaminated soil. The eggs hatch into larvae in the intestine. The larvae travel in the blood through the wall of the intestine to the lungs, up the windpipe, and are swallowed back into the small intestine. There they become adult worms.*

# ART THERAPY

In the aftermath of World War II, creative art began to be used on both sides of the Atlantic to help those who had undergone traumatic experiences deal with them and readjust to life. Spanning both conventional and complementary medicine, art therapy is now used by psychiatrists and psychotherapists worldwide as a technique in the diagnosis and treatment of mental and emotional disorders. It can also help people in emotional distress – for example, after a bereavement – providing therapeutic relief in expression through creative activities such as painting, drawing, and sculpting.

The expression of feelings in visual form has a long history, as ancient cave paintings attest. In the 19th century, Rudolf Steiner advocated the role of art in healing when developing anthroposophy. In the early 20th century, Carl Jung and Sigmund Freud ascribed to visual images the ability to reflect a patient's subconscious state, while other psychoanalysts, such as Anna Freud and Melanie Klein, later emphasized the value of creative art in childhood development.

After World War II, art therapy was used in the rehabilitation of war veterans. Under the guidance of art therapist Margaret Naumberg, it began to be taken seriously in the United States, where psychotherapy and other techniques based on Freudian theories were already well established. It is now widely practised in the United States, both for personal development and as a form of treatment for psychiatric disorders.

In the UK, art therapy developed in the 1940s, when artist Adrian Hill began to work informally with sanatorium patients. The British Association of Art Therapists was established in 1963, and there are now about 1,000 practitioners. A postgraduate Diploma of Art Therapy was recognized by the National Health Service in 1982, and art therapists were state-registered in 1997.

## Key principles

Patients are encouraged to express their feelings using materials such as paint, clay, crayons and fabric, or even magazines from which they can make a collage. They are not expected to produce a "good" work of art, but simply to give two- or three-dimensional expression to threatening or confused emotions. The act of releasing such emotions in the safe confines of the practitioner's consulting room is considered healing in itself, as the patient is able to overcome fear of self-expression and gain in confidence and self-esteem. Thoughts and emotions often surface visually in a work of art long before they might appear verbally in a conventional "talk" therapy, allowing issues to be addressed at a relatively early stage. Socially unacceptable emotions, such as jealousy or rage, can also be unearthed and confronted without fear of criticism.

Many people cope with mental and emotional problems by repressing them, mistakenly believing that they are taking firm control over their lives.

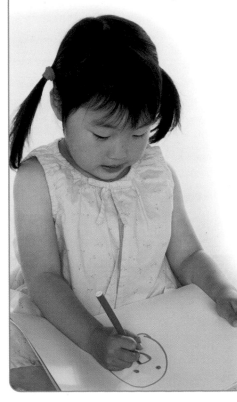

**For children, art therapy** *may be used as part of the treatment for emotional problems and learning difficulties. Sessions for children typically last about 30 minutes.*

In the early stages of art therapy, the challenge for such patients is to relinquish control sufficiently to create a therapeutically useful image.

Often, destructive impulses must be expressed before creativity and psychological insights can follow. Some patients need to make a mess, or to work carefully on an image only to destroy it, in order to achieve a breakthrough.

A further benefit of art therapy is that the work produced may contain symbols that can be interpreted by the practitioner, much as dreams may be analyzed in psychoanalysis.

Art therapy differs from psychoanalysis, however, in that it is the patient who takes the lead in interpretation, not the practitioner.

Art therapists believe that the individual holds the key to the symbols he or she produces, with the practitioner playing a supporting or guiding role.

## Evidence and research

Extensive casework in North America, the UK and Europe since the late 1980s has demonstrated the value of art therapy for a wide range of emotional and psychological disturbances, including psychotic illnesses, severe learning difficulties, eating disorders, and alcohol and drug abuse.

New areas currently being explored include relief in AIDS, Alzheimer's disease, and terminal illness.

## Medical opinion

Art therapy is extensively used in hospitals, prisons, and other institutions in the treatment of psychological disorders and addictions.

Most psychiatrists and doctors accept its role in treating learning difficulties and exploring the profound inner conflicts that arise when a life-threatening disease is diagnosed.

A

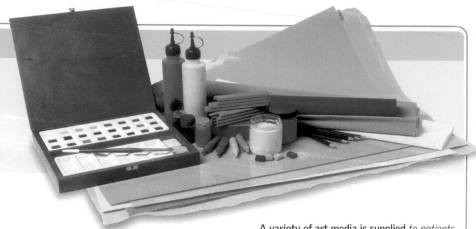

### Consulting a practitioner

Before therapy begins, the practitioner assesses your condition. Many patients, especially in the UK and Australia, may have been referred by a medical doctor. If this is the case, the practitioner reviews any notes or background information resulting from your previous treatment. He asks about your emotional problems, your life situation and your expectations from therapy. You, in turn, should take this opportunity to ask any questions you may have about the approach.

During a session, the practitioner avoids guiding you in an intrusive manner. He may respond to what you produce with questions and comments, in order to stimulate interpretation and further development.

Unexpected and disturbing images and associations may be made in the process, and the practitioner will help you explore the meanings uncovered and feelings that arise. If you are having difficulty with a particular medium, he may suggest changing to another or working with it in a different way.

Adult therapy sessions usually take place once a week and are 60–90 minutes long; children's sessions may last 30 minutes. A minimum of six months' treatment is recommended. Sessions may be one-to-one, or may take the form of group therapy, involving about 8–10 people. When working with a group, the practitioner might suggest theme-based exercises using dreams, relaxation, and visualization techniques.

Art therapy is sometimes practised in hospitals to supplement conventional psychotherapy. Up to three quarters of practitioners work in social services, prisons, and educational institutions. Some also work in private practice.

**A variety of art media is supplied** *to patients undergoing art therapy, including various paints, crayons, and papers. Each patient is allowed to choose a medium to suit them.*

### SELF HELP

Art therapy can be an ideal way to relax and allow problems to find a natural resolution. Talent or expertise is not important; the essential thing is to ignore the critical, inhibited part of yourself and let go. Choose the art media that most appeal to you. Some tips are given below:

● Begin by loosening up and allowing your intuition and spontaneity to surface. One way is to make initial sketches or paintings with your left hand if you are right-handed (or right hand if left-handed).

● Work quickly, without thinking about what you are doing. Put down the first shapes, forms and colours that come into your head.

● If you are uncomfortable with paints or clay, make a collage with images cut from newspapers and magazines.

● When finished, look carefully at your work. Do any symbols, shapes or colours hold significance? What feelings do they elicit? The meaning may not be clear, but try exploring these images in your artwork and see if they evolve.

## Aseptic technique

The creation of a germ-free environment to protect a patient from infection. Aseptic technique is used during surgery and other minor procedures, such as the insertion of a urinary catheter. It is also used during the care of people suffering from diseases in which the *immune system* is suppressed, such as *leukaemia*. Such conditions result in a weakening of the body's natural defences against infection.

All people who come in contact with the patient must scrub their hands and wear disposable gloves and masks and pre-sterilized gowns. Surgical instruments are sterilized in an autoclave. The patient's skin is cleaned with *antiseptic* solutions of, for example, iodine or *chlorhexidine*. In operating theatres, special ventilation systems purify the air. (See also *barrier nursing*; *isolation*.)

## Asperger's syndrome

A developmental disorder that is usually first recognized in childhood because of stilted speech, difficulties

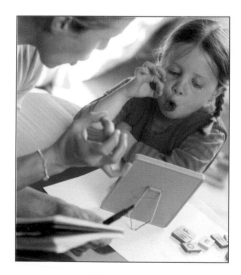

**Children who have developmental disorders**, *such as Asperger's syndrome, may be given special educational support to improve basic skills, such as social skills.*

with social interactions, and very specialized interests. Intelligence is normal or high.

Asperger's syndrome is one of a group of conditions known as pervasive developmental disorders; it is considered to be an *autism spectrum disorder* (a developmental disorder characterized by obsessive behaviour and impaired communication and social skills). Special educational support may be necessary, often within mainstream education. Asperger's syndrome is a lifelong condition.

## Aspergillosis

An infection caused by inhalation of spores of aspergillus, a fungus that grows in decaying vegetation. Aspergillus is harmless to healthy people but may proliferate in the lungs of people with *tuberculosis*. It can also worsen the symptoms of *asthma* and may produce serious, even fatal, infection in people with reduced immunity, such as those taking *immunosuppressant drugs*.

## Aspermia

See *azoospermia*.

## Asphyxia

The medical term for suffocation. Asphyxia may be caused by the obstruction of a large airway, usually by a foreign body (see *choking*), by insufficient oxygen in the surrounding air (as occurs when, for example, a closed plastic bag is put over the head), or by poisoning with a gas, such as carbon monoxide, that interferes with the uptake of oxygen into the blood.

The person initially breathes more rapidly and strongly to try to overcome the lack of oxygen in the blood. There is also an increase in heart rate and blood pressure. First-aid treatment is by clearing the airway of obstruction followed by *rescue*

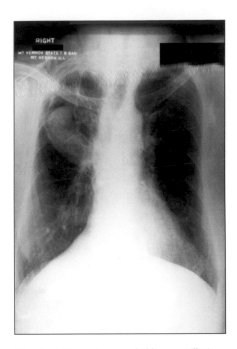

**This chest X-ray** *shows probable aspergillosis with an aspergilloma, or fungus ball, in the upper lobe of the right lung. Typically, the fungus lodges in the lung tissue in a cavity that has been caused by disease.*

breathing. Untreated asphyxia leads to death within a few minutes.

## Aspiration

The withdrawal of fluid or cells from the body by suction. The term also refers to the act of accidentally inhaling a foreign body, usually food or drink. If consciousness is impaired, for example by a head injury or excess alcohol intake, aspiration of the stomach contents is common.

Aspiration *biopsy* is the removal of cells or fluid, using a needle attached to a syringe, for examination. Aspiration biopsy is commonly used to obtain cells from

a fluid-filled cavity (such as a *breast cyst*). The procedure is also used to obtain cells from the bone marrow (see *bone marrow biopsy*), or from internal organs, when a fine needle is guided to the site of the biopsy by *CT scanning* or *ultrasound scanning*. (See also *aspiration pneumonia*.)

## Aspiration pneumonia

A form of pneumonia that results from accidental inhalation of vomit. Aspiration pneumonia usually occurs in people whose cough reflex is not functioning, such as those who have drunk excessive amounts of alcohol, taken certain illegal drugs, or suffered a head injury.

## Aspirin

A nonopioid *analgesic drug* (painkiller) that may be given in tablet or suppository form to treat disorders such as headache, menstrual pain, and muscle discomfort. Aspirin has an *anti-inflammatory* action. It also

**Aspirin is a nonopioid** *painkiller, used mainly for pain such as headache or menstrual pain. Aspirin also lowers fever and reduces inflammation.*

reduces fever and is included in some *cold remedies*.

In small doses, aspirin reduces the stickiness of platelets (blood particles involved in clotting). This has led to its use in preventing *thrombosis* (abnormal blood clots) in people at risk of developing *stroke* or *myocardial infarction* (heart attack) and as an initial treatment of chest pain that may be due to myocardial infarction. Aspirin may also reduce the risk of *colon cancer*.

In children, aspirin can cause *Reye's syndrome*, a rare but serious brain and liver disorder. For this reason, it should not be given to children under the age of 16 years, except on the advice of a doctor. Aspirin may cause irritation of the stomach lining, resulting in indigestion or nausea.

Prolonged use may cause bleeding from the stomach due to *gastric erosion* (disruption of the stomach lining) or *peptic ulcer*.

# Assay

The analysis or measurement of a substance to determine its presence or effects. A qualitative assay determines only whether or not a substance is present, whereas a quantitative assay determines the actual amount present.

Biological assays (known as bioassays) measure the response of an animal or organ to particular substances. Assays can be used, for example, to assess the effects of a drug or to measure hormone levels. (See also *immunoassay*.)

# Assisted conception

Treatment for *infertility* involving techniques that assist the fertilization and implantation of eggs. (See box, right).

# Association area

One of a number of areas in the cortex (outer layer) of the *brain* that are concerned with higher levels of mental

## ASSISTED CONCEPTION

Infertility treatments that involve mixing eggs and sperm outside the body include in-vitro fertilization (IVF), gamete intrafallopian transfer (GIFT), and zygote intrafallopian transfer (ZIFT). IVF is also used to treat some genetic disorders because the embryo can be tested for abnormalities before implantation.

### In-vitro fertilization
IVF may be performed if the cause of infertility cannot be determined or treated or if there is a blockage in a fallopian tube. Successful pregnancies occur in about 15 per cent of IVF attempts.

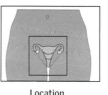

Location

**1** *Drugs are given to stimulate several eggs to mature in the ovaries. Under ultrasound guidance, the eggs are collected with a needle inserted through the vaginal wall.*

**2** *A sperm sample is combined with the collected eggs and the mixture is incubated for 48 hours at normal body temperature (37˚C or 98.6˚F) to allow fertilization to take place.*

Fallopian tubes

Follicles
These contain eggs ready for release

Hollow needle

Ultrasound probe
This guides the hollow needle to the eggs

Uterus

Ovary

Vagina

**3** *The fertilized eggs are introduced into the woman's uterus. Up to three eggs are injected through a thin tube that is fixed to a syringe and passed through the cervix. This procedure takes around 20 minutes. If one or more fertilized eggs implant, conception occurs.*

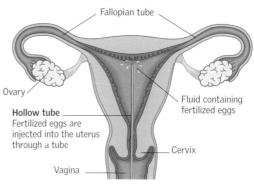

Fallopian tube

Ovary

Hollow tube
Fertilized eggs are injected into the uterus through a tube

Fluid containing fertilized eggs

Cervix

Vagina

### Other methods
The techniques GIFT and ZIFT may help couples who have unexplained infertility. In each method, eggs are collected as in IVF but are returned to the fallopian tube rather than the uterus. The success rate for both methods is 25–30 per cent.

### GIFT and ZIFT replacement methods
*In GIFT, eggs are mixed with sperm and then returned to the fallopian tube before fertilization. In ZIFT, the eggs are fertilized and returned to the fallopian tube.*

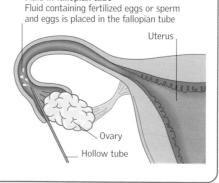

Fluid in fallopian tube
Fluid containing fertilized eggs or sperm and eggs is placed in the fallopian tube

Uterus

Ovary

Hollow tube

**A**

## YOUR BODY: ASSOCIATION AREAS

Large parts of the cerebral cortex are taken up by so-called "association areas", which analyse information received from the primary sensory sites. For example, a site called the primary auditory cortex registers basic information about the pitch and volume of sound (such as speech); Wernicke's area, part of the auditory association cortex, analyses speech so that it can be understood.

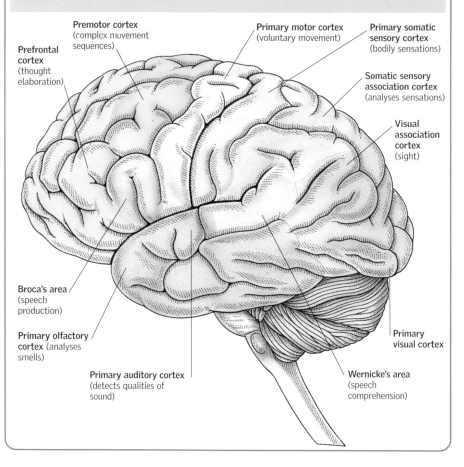

Prefrontal cortex (thought elaboration)

Premotor cortex (complex movement sequences)

Primary motor cortex (voluntary movement)

Primary somatic sensory cortex (bodily sensations)

Somatic sensory association cortex (analyses sensations)

Visual association cortex (sight)

Broca's area (speech production)

Primary olfactory cortex (analyses smells)

Primary auditory cortex (detects qualities of sound)

Primary visual cortex

Wernicke's area (speech comprehension)

activity. Association areas interpret information received from sensory areas and prompt appropriate responses, such as voluntary movement. (See box, above.)

## Associative aphasia

Also known as conductive aphasia, a form of *aphasia* (loss of language skills, including comprehension and/ or speech production) in which comprehension is normal, and the affected individual can write and speak, but he or she is unable to repeat what has been heard and cannot read aloud. Associative aphasia is caused by damage to a localized area in the brain, often as a result of a *stroke*.

## Astereognosis

The inability to recognize objects by touch when they are placed in the hand, even though there is no defect of sensation in the fingers or difficulty in holding the object. Astereognosis is either left- or right-sided; tactile recognition is normal on the other side. If both sides are affected, the condition is called tactile *agnosia*.

Astereognosis and tactile agnosia are caused by damage to parts of the *cerebrum* (the main mass of the brain) that are involved in recognition by touch. The conditions may occur as a result of a *stroke* or a *head injury*.

## Asthma

A lung disease in which there is intermittent narrowing of the *bronchi* (airways), causing shortness of breath, wheezing, and a cough.

The illness often starts in childhood but can develop at any age. At least one child in seven suffers from asthma, and the number affected has increased dramatically in recent years. Childhood asthma may be outgrown in about half of all cases.

During an asthma attack, the muscle in the walls of the airways contracts, causing narrowing. The lining of the airways also becomes swollen and inflamed, producing excess mucus that can block the smaller airways.

### TYPES AND CAUSES

In some people, an allergic response triggers the swelling and inflammation in the airways. This allergic type of asthma tends to occur in childhood, and it may develop in association with the allergic skin condition *eczema* or certain other allergic conditions such as hay fever (see *rhinitis, allergic*).

Continued on page 140

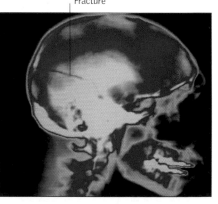

Fracture

**A colour-enhanced X-ray** *shows a skull fracture caused by a head injury. Such injuries may cause brain damage, which, in turn, may result in astereognosis.*

# ASTHMA

Asthma is inflammation and reversible constriction of the airways in the lungs, which causes recurrent episodes of breathlessness, wheezing, and sometimes a dry cough. It can be triggered by an allergic reactions to substances such as house dust or animal fur.

Metered-dose inhaler

Spacer

Drug suspended inside spacer

## Effect of asthma on the lungs

In asthma, the smaller bronchi and the bronchioles (smallest airways) become constricted, inflamed, and congested with mucus.

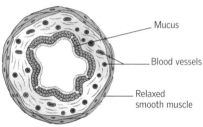

Mucus

Blood vessels

Relaxed smooth muscle

**Normal airway**
*Normally, the smooth muscle in the bronchial walls is relaxed, allowing a wide space for the passage of air.*

Inflammatory substances widen blood vessels

Increased mucus

Smooth muscle contracts

Inflammation and swelling

**In an asthma attack**
*During an attack of asthma, the muscle walls of the airways contract; increased mucus and inflamed tissues further narrow the airways.*

## Treating asthma

Drugs to prevent or treat asthma are often inhaled. Inhaled drugs reach the lungs quickly and have few side effects because only a small amount of drug enters the circulation. For treatment of a severe asthma attack, a nebulizer, which enables the delivery of large drug doses, may be used. Different devices are available for children.

Metered-dose inhaler

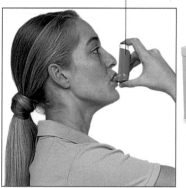

**Using an inhaler**
*Place the inhaler in front of the lips or in the mouth. Press the inhaler while breathing in deeply at the same time. Hold your breath for 10 seconds, then breathe out.*

## Spacers and inhalers

*A metered-dose inhaler (above) delivers a precise dose when the inhaler is pressed. A spacer can be used to hold the dose before it is inhaled. Spacers allow the drug to be inhaled over several breaths.*

**Drug chamber**
The drug is dissolved in 3–5 ml of fluid

Mouthpiece

**Tube**
This delivers compressed air

Compressor

**Using a nebulizer**
*A nebulizer creates a fine mist of drugs by forcing compressed air or oxygen through a liquid dose of the drug. The drug in mist form is then inhaled, through either a mouthpiece or a face mask.*

A

## REDUCING THE RISK OF ASTHMA ATTACKS

- Do not smoke and try to avoid polluted or smoky atmospheres. Do not allow people to smoke in the house.

- Take regular exercise to improve your stamina. Swimming is a particularly beneficial form of exercise. Avoid exercising outside when it is cold.

- If your attacks are triggered by stress, practise relaxation exercises.

- Avoid substances that are likely to provoke an allergic response; do not keep furry animals as pets if you are allergic to them.

- Always carry an inhaler, and take medication with you on holiday.

- Dust furniture using a damp cloth and vacuum carpets regularly.

- Enclose mattresses in plastic covers.

- If pollen is a problem, keep windows closed, especially while grass is releasing pollen, and use an air purifier.

- Do not use fluffy, dust-collecting blankets and make sure pillows and duvets contain artificial fibres.

- Avoid products that have strong odours, such as air fresheners, mothballs and perfumes.

## MONITORING YOUR ASTHMA

The best way to monitor your asthma is with a peak flow meter, which is used every morning and evening to measure the maximum rate at which you can exhale in litres per minute. The reading indicates whether your airways are narrowed. Plotted on a chart, your peak flow results show how effectively your asthma is being controlled. You can then adjust your treatment, following advice given to you previously by your doctor.

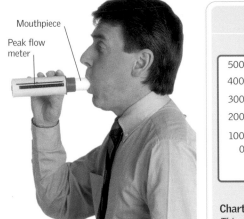

Mouthpiece

Peak flow meter

**Using a peak flow meter**
*You should take a full breath in, seal your lips around the mouthpiece, and exhale as hard as you can. The pointer on the side of the meter shows your peak flow result.*

### RESULTS

**Charting your peak flow**
*This chart shows twice-daily peak flow readings with marked variations between the morning and evening readings. These variations indicate that the asthma is poorly controlled.*

Susceptibility to these conditions frequently runs in families.

Some substances are known to trigger attacks of allergic asthma (see *allergens*). These include pollen, house-dust mites, mould, feathers, and dander (tiny scales) and saliva from furry animals such as cats and dogs. Rarely, certain foods, such as milk, eggs, nuts, and wheat, provoke an allergic asthmatic reaction. Some people with asthma are sensitive to *aspirin*, and taking it may trigger an attack.

When asthma starts in adulthood, there are usually no identifiable allergic triggers. The first attack is sometimes brought on by a respiratory tract infection, stress, or anxiety.

In some cases, a substance that is inhaled regularly in the work environment can result in the development of asthma in a previously healthy person. This is known as occupational asthma, and it is one of the few occupational lung diseases that are still increasing in incidence.

There are currently about 200 substances used in the workplace that are known to trigger symptoms of asthma, including glues, resins, latex, and some chemicals, especially isocyanate chemicals used in spray painting. However, occupational asthma can be difficult to diagnose because a person may be regularly exposed to a particular trigger substance for weeks, months, or even years before the symptoms of asthma begin to appear.

Factors that can provoke attacks in a person with asthma include cold air, exercise, smoke, and occasionally emotional factors such as stress and anxiety. Although industrial pollution and exhaust emission from motor vehicles do not normally cause asthma, they do appear to worsen symptoms in people who already have the disorder.

Pollution in the atmosphere may also trigger asthma in people who are susceptible.

### SYMPTOMS

Asthma attacks can vary in severity from mild breathlessness to *respiratory failure*.

The main symptoms are wheezing, breathlessness, dry cough, and a tightness in the chest. In a severe attack, breathing becomes increasingly difficult, resulting in a low level of oxygen in the blood. This causes *cyanosis* (a bluish discoloration) of the face, particularly of the lips. Left untreated, such attacks can be fatal.

### TREATMENT

There is no cure for asthma, but attacks can be prevented to a large extent if a particular allergen can be identified and consequently avoided.

Treatment involves inhaled *bronchodilator drugs* (sometimes known as relievers) to widen the airways, thereby relieving symptoms. When symptoms occur frequently, or are severe, inhaled *corticosteroids* are also prescribed. These drugs (also known as preventers) are used continuously to prevent attacks by reducing inflammation in the airways.

Other drug treatments include *sodium cromoglicate* and nedocromil sodium, both of which are useful in the prevention of exercise-induced asthma. The use of a *leukotriene receptor antagonist* in combination with a corticosteroid drug may enable the required dose of corticosteroid to be reduced. *Theophylline* or the inhaled *anticholinergic drug* ipratropium bromide may also be used as broncho-dilators. An asthma attack that has not responded to treatment with a bronchodilator needs immediate assessment and treatment in hospital.

A

## HAVING A VISION TEST

You should have your vision tested by a qualified optician or ophthalmologist every two years, especially if you are over the age of 40. The most common tests assess the acuity (sharpness) of your distance vision and your ability to focus on near objects, as well as checking for other common conditions such as astigmatism. The tests also show which corrective lenses, if any, you need. Additional tests for specific eye disorders, such as glaucoma, may be performed, depending on your age and medical history.

**Phoropter**
This device can hold different lenses in front of each eye, allowing the eyes to be tested separately

**Adjustable arm**
The position of the trial frame is adjusted to your height

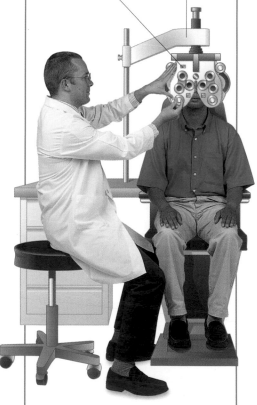

## Asthma, cardiac

Breathing difficulty in which *broncho-spasm* (narrowing of the airways) and wheezing occur as a result of fluid accumulation in the lungs (*pulmonary oedema*). Cardiac asthma is usually due to reduced pumping efficiency of the left side of the heart (see *heart failure*) and is not true asthma. Treatment is with *diuretic drugs* or other drugs for heart failure.

## Astigmatism

A condition in which the front surface of the *cornea* does not conform to the normal "spherical" curve, even though the eye is perfectly healthy. Because the cornea is unevenly curved, it refracts (bends) the light rays that strike it to differing degrees. The *lens* is then unable to bring all the rays into focus on the light-sensitive *retina*. A minor degree of astigmatism is normal and does not require correction. More severe astigmatism causes blurring of lines at a certain angle and does require correction.

### DIAGNOSIS AND TREATMENT

Astigmatism can usually be diagnosed with standard vision tests (see box, left). It can be corrected by using special "cylindrical" glasses that can be framed at a precise angle; contact lenses that can give an even spherical surface for focusing; or by undergoing *laser treatment* on the cornea.

## Astringents

### COMMON DRUGS

• Aluminium acetate • Potassium permanganate • Silver nitrate • Zinc sulphate

Substances that causes tissue to dry and shrink by reducing its ability to absorb water. Astringents are widely used in *antiperspirants* and to promote healing of broken or inflamed skin. They are also used in some eye or ear preparations. Astringents may cause burning or stinging when applied.

## Astrocytoma

A type of cancerous brain tumour. Astrocytomas are the most common type of *glioma*, a tumour that arises from the glial (supporting) cells within the nervous system.

Astrocytomas most commonly develop in the cerebrum (the main mass of the brain) and are classified in four grades (I to IV) according to their rate of growth and malignancy. A grade I astrocytoma is a slow-growing tumour that may spread widely throughout the brain but may be present for many years before causing symptoms. The most severe and fast-growing type is called *glioblastoma multiforme* (a grade IV astrocytoma).

Symptoms are similar to those of other types of brain tumour. Diagnostic tests include *CT scanning* or *MRI*. Treatment is with surgery as well as, in some cases, *radiotherapy*.

## Asymptomatic

A medical term meaning without *symptoms* (indications of illness noticed only by the patient). For example, *hypertension* (high blood pressure) is often asymptomatic and is usually discovered during a routine blood pressure test, while *diabetes mellitus* is often diagnosed from a routine blood or urine test. Most disorders have no symptoms in their early stages. In the case of *cancer*, much effort has been made to devise screening tests to detect tumours at their early, asymptomatic, stage. (See also *sign*.)

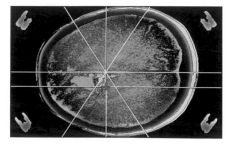

**A CT scan of the brain** *reveals a tumour – a high-grade astrocytoma – shown here in green..*

# Ataxia

Incoordination and clumsiness that may affect balance and gait (see *walking*), limb and eye movements, and/or speech.

## CAUSES

Ataxia may be the result of damage to the *cerebellum* (the part of the brain concerned with coordination) or to nerve pathways in the *brainstem* (a stalk of nerve tissue linking the brain to the *spinal cord*) and/or spinal cord. Possible causes include injury to the brain or spinal cord.

In adults, ataxia may be caused by *alcohol intoxication*; a *stroke* or *brain tumour* affecting the cerebellum or brainstem; a disease of the balance organ in the ear; or *multiple sclerosis* or other types of nerve degeneration.

In children, causes include acute infection, brain tumours, and the inherited condition *Friedreich's ataxia*.

## SYMPTOMS

Symptoms of ataxia depend on the site of damage within the nervous system, although a lurching, unsteady gait is common to most forms.

In addition, damage to certain parts of the brain may cause *nystagmus* (jerky eye movements) and slurred speech.

## DIAGNOSIS AND TREATMENT

*CT scanning* or *MRI* (techniques that produce cross-sectional or three-dimensional images of body structures) may be used to determine the cause of ataxia. Treatment of the condition depends on the cause.

# Atelectasis

Collapse of part or all of a *lung* caused by obstruction of the bronchus (the main air passage through the lung) or the bronchioles (smaller air passages). When obstruction occurs, air already in the lung cannot be breathed out and is therefore absorbed into the blood, leading to the collapse of all or part of the lung. After collapsing, the lung loses its elasticity and cannot take in air; consequently, the blood passing through it can no longer absorb oxygen or dispose of carbon dioxide.

In an adult, atelectasis is not normally life-threatening because unaffected parts of the lung and/or the other lung can compensate for the loss of function in the collapsed area. However, when a newborn baby's lung collapses, the baby's life is at risk.

**This CT scan** *through a patient's chest shows collapse (atelectasis) of the right lung, which is filled with fluid and unable to expand properly. Healthy tissue in the lung has shrunk as a result.*

## CAUSES

Obstruction of a bronchus or bronchiole may be caused by the accumulation of mucus. This buildup of mucus most commonly occurs in a baby at birth; in people with asthma; after an abdominal or chest operation that has made coughing difficult because of pain; in certain infections such as *pertussis* (whooping cough) in children or chronic *bronchitis* (bronchial inflammation) in adults.

Obstruction may also result from an accidentally inhaled foreign body, a tumour in the lung, or enlarged *lymph nodes* (which occur in *tuberculosis*, some other lung infections, or certain forms of *cancer*) exerting pressure on the airway. The collapsed lung may become infected.

## SYMPTOMS

The main symptom of atelectasis is shortness of breath. There may also be a cough and chest pain, depending on the underlying cause

## DIAGNOSIS AND TREATMENT

Atelectasis can be diagnosed by *chest X-ray*, and treatment is aimed at removing the cause of the blockage. The treatment may include *physiotherapy* or *bronchoscopy*, a procedure that involves removal of the blockage using a rigid or flexible viewing tube (see *endoscope*). If the obstruction can be removed, the lung should reinflate normally.

# Atenolol

A *beta-blocker drug* that is commonly used to treat *hypertension* (high blood pressure), angina pectoris (chest pain caused by an impaired blood supply to the heart muscle), and certain types of *arrhythmia* (irregular heartbeat) in which the heart beats too rapidly.

# Atheroma

Fatty deposits on the inner lining of an artery that occur in *atherosclerosis*

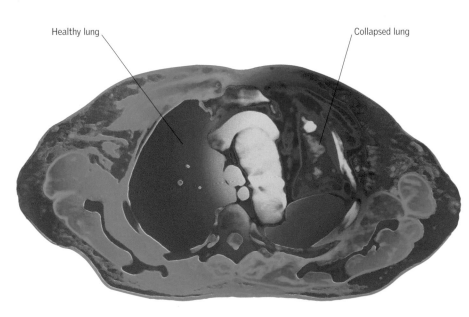

Healthy lung          Collapsed lung

and restrict blood flow. The deposits are also known as atheromatous plaques.

# Atherosclerosis

The accumulation of *cholesterol* and other fatty substances (lipids) in the walls of arteries, causing the arteries to narrow (see boxes right).

Atherosclerosis can affect arteries in any area of the body and is a major cause of stroke, heart attack (see *myocardial infarction*), and poor circulation in the legs.

The arteries become narrowed when fatty substances carried in the blood accumulate on the inside lining of the arteries and form yellow deposits known as atheromatous plaques. These deposits restrict the blood flow

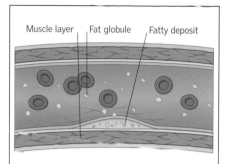

**Early atherosclerosis**
*The arteries begin to slowly narrow when fatty substances that are carried in the blood accumulate on the lining of the arteries.*

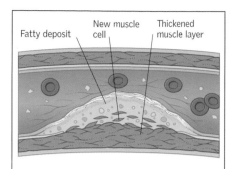

**Advanced atherosclerosis**
*Over time, the muscle layer of the artery wall (under the fatty deposit) thickens, narrowing the artery and restricting blood flow even more.*

through the arteries. In addition, the muscle layer of the artery wall becomes thickened, which narrows the artery even further. Platelets (tiny blood cells that are responsible for

blood clotting) may collect in clumps on the surface of the deposits and initiate the formation of blood clots. A large clot may completely block the artery, resulting in the organ it

## ARTERIAL DEGENERATION IN ATHEROSCLEROSIS

Atherosclerosis is narrowing of the arteries due to plaques of atheroma on their inner linings. The plaques are composed mainly of fats, deposited from the bloodstream, that disrupt normal blood flow through the artery. Men are affected earlier than women because premenopausal women are protected by natural oestrogen hormones.

### RISK FACTORS

- Cigarette smoking
- Hypertension (high blood pressure)
- Male gender
- Obesity
- Physical inactivity
- Diabetes mellitus
- Heredity
- High blood cholesterol

**Plaques**
*The fatty deposits known as plaques consist of a fatty core topped by a fibrous cap. If blood turbulence roughens the surface of the plaques, platelets and blood cells can collect, creating a blood clot that may block the artery completely. This may lead to embolism, in which a fragment of the clot breaks off and travels in the bloodstream to another site.*

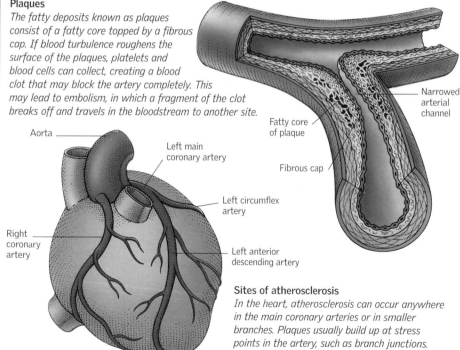

Narrowed arterial channel

Fatty core of plaque

Fibrous cap

Aorta

Left main coronary artery

Left circumflex artery

Left anterior descending artery

Right coronary artery

**Sites of atherosclerosis**
*In the heart, atherosclerosis can occur anywhere in the main coronary arteries or in smaller branches. Plaques usually build up at stress points in the artery, such as branch junctions.*

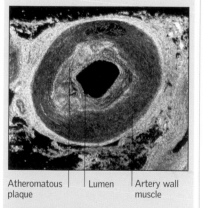

Atheromatous plaque | Lumen | Artery wall muscle

**Atherosclerosis**
*The artery shown here has an atheromatous (fibrous and fatty) plaque deposit on its inner wall. The lumen (channel) has been narrowed, impeding blood flow.*

A

supplies being deprived of oxygen. A complete blockage in a coronary artery can cause a sudden, often fatal, heart attack.

### CAUSES

The risk of developing atherosclerosis is determined largely by the level of cholesterol in the bloodstream, which depends on dietary and genetic factors. Atherosclerosis is more common in developed countries, where most people eat a diet high in fat. Some disorders such as *diabetes mellitus* can be associated with a high cholesterol level, regardless of diet.

### SYMPTOMS

Atherosclerosis usually produces no symptoms in its early stages. As the condition progresses, symptoms occur as a result of reduced, or total absence of, blood supply to the organs supplied by the affected arteries.

Partial blockage of the coronary arteries (which supply the heart muscle) may produce symptoms such as the chest pain of angina pectoris. Narrowing of the arteries supplying blood to the brain may cause *transient ischaemic attacks* (symptoms and signs of a *stroke* that last for less than 24 hours) and episodes of dizziness.

Intermittent *claudication* (a cramplike pain on walking) is often the first symptom of atherosclerosis in the leg arteries.

If the condition is associated with an inherited lipid disorder (see *hyperlipidaemias*), fatty deposits may develop on tendons or as visible lumps under the skin.

### DIAGNOSIS AND TREATMENT

Blood flow through an artery can be investigated by *angiography* (X-rays taken after injection of a *radiopaque* substance) or *Doppler* ultrasound scanning.

The best treatment for atherosclerosis is to prevent it from progressing by the maintenance of a healthy lifestyle. This includes adoption of a low-fat diet, not smoking, regular

## YOUR BODY: BASAL GANGLIA

These masses, or nuclei, of grey matter, which include the lentiform and caudate nuclei, are located deep in the brain. Damage to the basal ganglia can cause athetosis and chorea, conditions which affect movement.

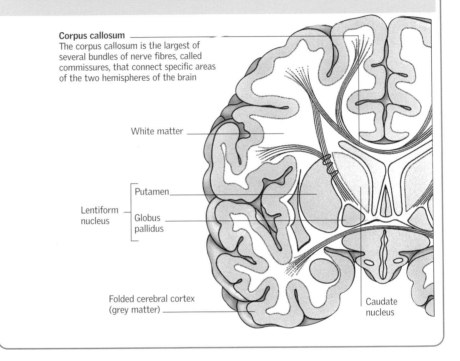

**Corpus callosum**
The corpus callosum is the largest of several bundles of nerve fibres, called commissures, that connect specific areas of the two hemispheres of the brain

White matter

Putamen

Lentiform nucleus

Globus pallidus

Folded cerebral cortex (grey matter)

Caudate nucleus

exercise, and maintenance of the recommended weight for height. These measures lead to a reduced risk of developing significant atherosclerosis.

Those individuals found to have high blood cholesterol levels but who are otherwise in good health will be advised to adopt a low-fat diet.

They may also be given drugs that decrease blood cholesterol levels (see *lipid-lowering drugs*). For people who have had a heart attack, research has shown that there may be a benefit in lowering blood cholesterol levels, even if the level is within the average range for healthy people.

People with atherosclerosis and those at risk may be prescribed a drug such as *aspirin* to reduce the risk of blood clots forming on the damaged artery lining.

Surgical treatment of atherosclerosis, such as coronary angioplasty (see *angioplasty, balloon*), may be recommended for those people

thought to be at high risk of severe complications. If blood flow to the heart is severely obstructed, a *coronary artery bypass* may be carried out to restore blood flow.

## Athetosis

A disorder of the nervous system that is characterized by involuntary slow, writhing movements, most often of the face, head, neck, and limbs. These movements commonly include facial grimacing, with contortions of the mouth. There may also be difficulty in balancing and walking.

Athetosis tends to be combined with *chorea* (involuntary irregular, jerky movements). Both athetosis and chorea arise from damage to the *basal ganglia* (see box, above), clusters of nerve cells in the brain that control movement.

Causes of athetosis include brain damage prior to or at birth (see

# SELF HELP: ATHLETE'S FOOT AND JOCK ITCH

These are common fungal infections. Athlete's foot affects the skin between the toes, making it cracked, sore, and itchy with peeling areas. It may spread to the soles and toenails. Jock itch is an itchy, scaly, red rash in the groin, more common in men. Both infections thrive in warm, sweaty conditions. You can catch them from contact with an infected person or sharing items such as towels and footwear.

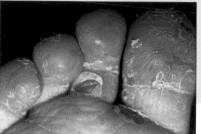

Athlete's foot between the toes

## WHAT YOU CAN DO YOURSELF

Both infections are easy to treat yourself. Keep using the good hygiene practices outlined below to help prevent fungal infections recurring.

### Athlete's foot

- Treat the infection with an antifungal cream and/or powder (see drug remedies, right).

- Wash your feet twice daily, making sure you dry thoroughly between your toes afterwards.

- Use a separate towel just for drying your feet, and launder the towel frequently.

- Wear socks made from natural fibres and change them at least once a day. Women should avoid wearing tights and stockings, especially those that cramp the feet.

- Wear well-ventilated shoes made from natural rather than synthetic materials; open-toed sandals are particularly good.

- Wear flip-flops when walking around communal changing areas, such as at swimming baths.

### Jock itch

- Apply an antifungal treatment to the infected area (see drug remedies, right).

- Wash your groin regularly, drying it thoroughly but avoiding chafing. Use a separate towel to dry this area, and launder the towel frequently.

- Don't wear tight-filling trousers or underwear, or underwear made from synthetic fabrics. Cotton pants or boxer shorts are best. Change them daily.

## DRUG REMEDIES

Antifungal drugs, such as clotrimazole, miconazole, or terbinafine, are used to treat athlete's foot and jock itch. They are available from pharmacies as a cream or a fine powder spray, which is usually easier to apply. Most are recommended to be applied twice daily.

The infection should start to clear up within a week, although it may take several weeks longer before it disappears completely. To treat athlete's foot, you can dust inside your socks and shoes with antifungal foot powder, also available from pharmacies.

## SEEK MEDICAL ADVICE

Arrange to see your doctor if:
- The affected area becomes hot and red, or starts weeping
- The infection does not clear up after you have tried self-help treatment

**Powder spray**
*Apply the powder after washing and drying your feet carefully. Spray generously, paying particular attention to areas between the toes.*

## ATRIAL FIBRILLATION

This is the most common type of rapid, irregular heart rate. It most often occurs in people over 60, and up to one in twenty of very elderly people in the UK may be affected by it. Your doctor may suspect atrial fibrillation if you have a fast, irregular pulse. To confirm the diagnosis, you will have electrocardiography (ECG) to check your heartbeat.

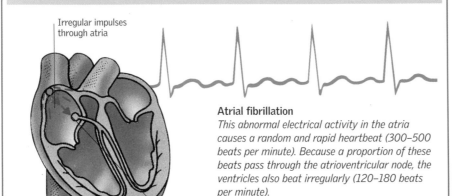

Irregular impulses through atria

**Atrial fibrillation**
*This abnormal electrical activity in the atria causes a random and rapid heartbeat (300–500 beats per minute). Because a proportion of these beats pass through the atrioventricular node, the ventricles also beat irregularly (120–180 beats per minute).*

Variable blockage at atrioventricular (AV) node

cerebral palsy), *encephalitis* (brain infection), degenerative disorders such as *Huntington's disease*, or as a side effect of *phenothiazine drugs* or *levodopa*.

If drug treatment is the cause of the condition, the abnormal movements may stop when the drug is withdrawn.

## Athlete's foot

A common condition in which the skin between the toes becomes itchy and sore and may crack, peel, or blister.

### CAUSES
Athlete's foot is usually the result of a fungal infection known medically as

tinea pedis, but the condition may also be caused by bacteria.

Because the fungi thrive in humid conditions, athlete's foot is more common in people with particularly sweaty feet and those who wear shoes and socks made from synthetic fibres, which do not absorb sweat.

### TREATMENT
Self-treatment with topical *antifungal drugs* is usually effective and should be combined with careful foot hygiene. (See box, previous page.)

## Atlas

The topmost cervical *vertebra* in the human *spine*. The atlas is attached to and supports the skull.

A pivot joint attaching the atlas to the second cervical vertebra, the *axis*, allows the atlas to rotate, thereby turning the head from side to side.

## Atony

Loss of tension in a muscle, so that it is completely flaccid. Atony can occur in some nervous system disorders or after injury to nerves. For example, the arm muscles may become atonic after injury to the *brachial plexus* (nerve roots in the neck passing into the arm).

## Atopic eczema

Atopic *eczema* is the most common form of eczema (an inflammatory skin condition). It usually begins in infancy but may flare up during adolescence and adulthood. The cause of atopic eczema is unknown, but people with *atopy* (a predisposition to allergic reactions) are more susceptible.

## Atopy

A predisposition to various allergic reactions (see *allergy*). Atopic

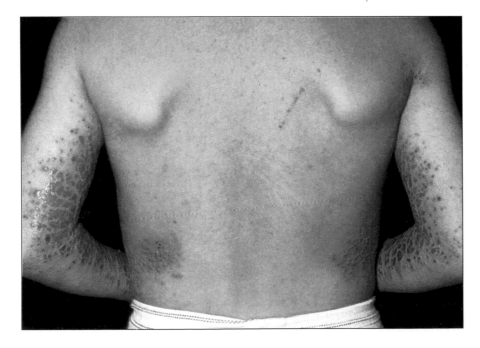

**This picture shows** *chronic atopic eczema on an arm, with redness, crusting, and thickening and hardening of the skin.*

individuals have a tendency to suffer from one or more allergic disorders, such as *asthma*, *eczema*, *urticaria* (nettle rash), and allergic *rhinitis* (hay fever). The mechanism that underlies the predisposition is unclear, but atopy seems to run in families.

# ATP

An abbreviation for the compound adenosine triphosphate, the principal energy-carrying chemical in the body. (See also *ADP*; *metabolism*.)

# Atresia

*Congenital* (present from birth) absence or severe narrowing of a body opening or tubular organ due to a failure of development in the uterus. Examples are *biliary atresia*, in which the bile ducts between the liver and duodenum are absent; *oesophageal atresia*, in which the oesophagus comes to a blind end; and anal atresia (see *anus, imperforate*), in which the anal canal is shut off. Most forms of atresia require surgical correction early in life.

# Atrial fibrillation

A type of abnormality of the heartbeat (see *arrhythmia, cardiac*) in which the atria (see *atrium*), the upper chambers of the heart, beat irregularly and very rapidly. The *ventricles* (the heart's lower chambers) also beat irregularly but at a slower rate. As a result, the pumping ability of the heart is reduced. (See box, left.)

## CAUSES
Atrial fibrillation can occur in almost any longstanding heart disease, but it is most often associated with *heart-valve disorders* or *coronary artery disease*.

## SYMPTOMS AND SIGNS
Sudden onset of atrial fibrillation can cause *palpitations* (awareness of a fast heartbeat), angina pectoris (chest pain as due to impaired blood supply to the heart muscle), or breathlessness. The inefficient pumping action of the heart reduces the output of blood into the circulation. Blood clots may form in the atria and may enter the bloodstream and lodge in an artery (see *embolism*).

## DIAGNOSIS AND TREATMENT
Diagnosis of atrial fibrillation is confirmed by an *ECG*, which shows the electrical activity of the heart.

Digoxin or *beta-blocker drugs* may be given to control the heart rate. If the atrial fibrillation is of recent onset, it may be reversed by *defibrillation* (the application of a short electric shock to the heart). In most cases, *anticoagulant drugs* or *aspirin* are also given to reduce the risk of an embolism occurring.

# Atrial flutter

A type of abnormality of the heartbeat (see *arrhythmia, cardiac*) in which the atria (see *atrium*), the heart's upper chambers beat regularly but very rapidly. Symptoms and treatment of atrial flutter are the same as for *atrial fibrillation*.

# Atrial natriuretic peptide

A substance that is produced in special cells in the muscular wall of the atria (see *atrium*), the upper chambers of the heart. Atrial natriuretic peptide is released into the bloodstream in response to swelling of the atrial muscle due, for example, to *heart failure* or *hypertension* (high blood pressure).

Atrial natriuretic peptide increases the amount of sodium excreted in the urine. Sodium draws water out with it, which decreases the volume of the blood, thereby reducing blood pressure.

Children who have congenital heart disorders that result in heart disease (see *heart disease, congenital*) possess high levels of atrial natriuretic peptide. Following successful surgery to correct the heart abnormality, the levels of atrial natriuretic peptide fall.

## ATRIAL SEPTAL DEFECT

A hole in the septum, the wall that separates the atria and ventricles (heart chambers), allows oxygenated blood mixed with deoxygenated blood to flow to the lungs (which should receive deoxygenated blood only). The defect is often found in children with Down's syndrome.

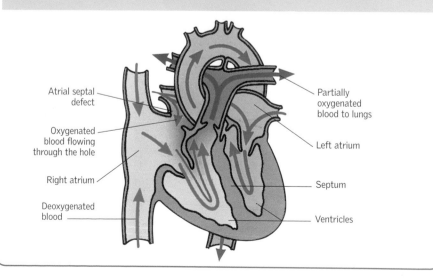

Atrial septal defect

Oxygenated blood flowing through the hole

Right atrium

Deoxygenated blood

Partially oxygenated blood to lungs

Left atrium

Septum

Ventricles

# Atrial septal defect (ASD)

A congenital (present from birth) heart abnormality (see *heart disease, congenital*) in which there is a hole in the dividing wall (see *septal defect*) between the heart's two upper chambers, or atria (see *atrium*), allowing deoxygenated blood to mix with oxygenated blood and flow to the lungs. (See box, on previous page.)

# Atrioventricular block

A type of *heart block*.

# Atrioventricular node

A small knot of specialized muscle cells in the right *atrium* (upper chamber) of the heart. Electrical impulses from the *sinoatrial node* (a cluster of muscle cells that act as the heart's natural pacemaker) pass through the atrioventricular node and along conducting fibres to the *ventricles* (the lower chambers of the heart), causing them to contract and pump blood around the body.

# Atrium

Also known as an auricle, either of the two (right and left) upper chambers of the *heart*. The atria open directly into the *ventricles* (the lower chambers of the heart). Deoxygenated blood from the body enters the right atrium through the *venae cavae*. Oxygenated blood from the lungs enters the left atrium through the *pulmonary veins*.

**A child with attention deficit hyperactivity disorder** *is likely to be restless, inattentive, and unable to sit still for more than a few moments.*

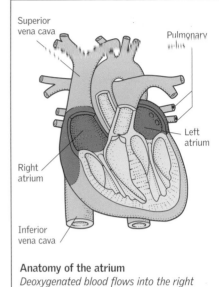

**Anatomy of the atrium**
*Deoxygenated blood flows into the right atrium through the venae cavae; oxygenated blood flows into the left atrium via the pulmonary veins.*

# Atrophy

The wasting away or shrinkage of a normally developed tissue or organ that results from a reduction in the size or number of its cells.

Atrophy is commonly caused by disuse (such as when a limb has been immobilized in a plaster cast) or inadequate cell nutrition as a result of poor blood circulation. Atrophy may also occur during prolonged illness, when the body needs to use up the protein reserves in the muscles. In some circumstances, atrophy is a normal process (as in ovarian atrophy, for example, which occurs in women who have passed the *menopause*.

# Atropine

An *anticholinergic drug* that is derived from the deadly-nightshade plant (see *belladonna*). Atropine is used to dilate the pupil in eye conditions such as iritis (inflammation of the iris) and *corneal ulcer*. It is also used in young children, in the form of eye-drops, to dilate (widen) the *pupil* for examination.

Atropine was often given (by injection) as a *premedication* before a

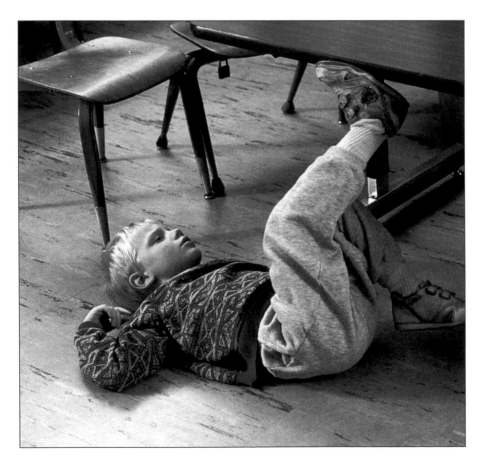

## AUDIOMETRY

This test measures how loud a sound has to be for you to hear it. Sounds of varying frequency are transmitted to one ear at a time through headphones. For each frequency, the volume is increased until you hear it, and the results are recorded. The test is repeated with a speaker held against a bone behind the ear.

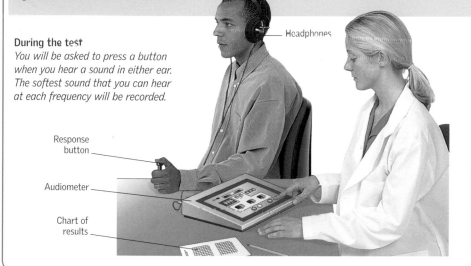

**During the test**
*You will be asked to press a button when you hear a sound in either ear. The softest sound that you can hear at each frequency will be recorded.*

Headphones

Response button

Audiometer

Chart of results

### AUDIOMETRY TRACE

This trace is from a person with normal hearing in the left ear and sensorineural hearing loss in the right. At higher frequencies, the right ear can detect sound only if the sound level is much higher than normal.

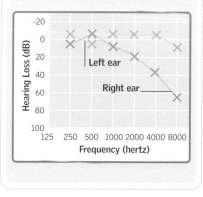

general anaesthetic (see *anaesthesia, general*) to reduce secretions from the lungs, but it is now rarely used for this purpose. It is used as emergency treatment for *bradycardia* (abnormally slow heartbeat) and is also sometimes prescribed for its anticholinergic effects; it is combined with an *antidiarrhoeal drug* to relieve the abdominal cramps that accompany diarrhoea.

Side effects include dry mouth, blurred vision, retention of urine, and, in the elderly, confusion. Atropine eye-drops are rarely given to adults because they cause disturbance of vision that lasts for two to three weeks and may precipitate acute *glaucoma* in susceptible people.

# Attention deficit hyperactivity disorder (ADHD)

A behavioural disorder in which a child has a consistently high level of activity and/or difficulty in attending to tasks.

Attention deficit hyperactivity, or hyperkinetic, disorder affects up to five per cent of children in the UK.

The disorder, which is more common in boys, should not be confused with the normal boisterous conduct of a healthy child. Children with ADHD show abnormal patterns of behaviour over a period of time. An affected child is likely to be constantly restless, unable to sit still for more than a few moments, inattentive, and impulsive.

### CAUSES

The causes of ADHD are not fully understood, but the disorder often runs in families, which suggests that genetic factors may be involved. ADHD is not, as popularly believed, a result of poor parenting or abuse.

### SYMPTOMS AND SIGNS

Symptoms of the condition develop in early childhood, usually between the ages of three and seven, and may include the inability to finish tasks; inability to concentrate in class; a short attention span; difficulty in

following instructions; a tendency to talk excessively, frequently interrupting other people; difficulty in waiting or taking turns; inability to play alone, quietly; and physical impulsiveness.

Children with ADHD may have difficulty in forming friendships. Self-esteem is often low because an affected child is frequently scolded and criticized.

### TREATMENT AND OUTLOOK

Treatment of ADHD includes behaviour modification techniques, both at home and at school. In some children, avoidance of certain foods or food additives seems to reduce symptoms. In severe cases, *stimulant drugs*, usually *methylphenidate*, may be prescribed. Paradoxically, the use of stimulant drugs in the treatment of ADHD reduces hyperactivity and improves concentration.

In general, the condition improves by adolescence but may be followed by antisocial behaviour and *drug abuse* or *substance abuse*.

## YOUR BODY: AUDITORY NERVE

Part of the vestibulochlear nerve, the auditory nerve (sometimes also known as the acoustic nerve) transmits nerve impulses from the cochlea (the receptor for hearing) in the inner ear to the brain.

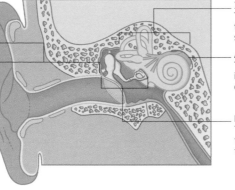

**Outer ear**
The pinna and ear canal are parts of the outer ear

**Inner ear**
This contains the cochlea and semicircular canals

**Auditory nerve**
This transmits nerve impulses from the cochlea to the brain

**Middle ear**
The auditory ossicles transmit sound across this space

## Attenuated

A term used to refer to micro-organisms that have been treated to reduce their ability to cause disease. Attenuated organisms are used in some *vaccines*.

## Atypical

A term used to describe something that is not the usual type or that does not fit into the usual pattern. The atypical presentation of a disease or disorder is one in which the early symptoms and signs differ from those that normally occur, which may make diagnosis of the condition more difficult.

## Audiogram

A graph that is produced as a result of *audiometry* (measurement of the sense of hearing). An audiogram shows the hearing threshold (the minimum audible decibel level) for each of a range of sound frequencies.

## Audiology

The study of hearing, especially impaired hearing.

## Audiometry

Measurement of the sense of hearing. The term audiometry often refers to *hearing tests* in which a machine is used to produce sounds of a defined intensity (loudness) and frequency (pitch), and in which the hearing in each ear is measured over the full range of normally audible sounds. (See also *impedance audiometry*.)

## Auditory nerve

The part of the *vestibulocochlear nerve* (the eighth *cranial nerve*) concerned with hearing. The auditory nerve is also known as the acoustic nerve. (See box, above.)

## Aura

A peculiar "warning" sensation that precedes or marks the onset of a *migraine* attack or a seizure in *epilepsy*.

A migraine attack may be preceded by a feeling of elation, excessive energy, or drowsiness; thirst or a craving for sweet foods may develop. A migraine may also be heralded by flashing lights before the eyes, blurred or tunnel vision, or difficulty in speaking. There may also be weakness, numbness, or tingling in one half of the body. As these symptoms subside, the migraine headache begins.

An epileptic aura may occur as a distorted perception, such as a hallucinatory smell or sound or a sensation of movement in a part of the body.

One type of attack (in people who have *temporal lobe epilepsy*) is often preceded by a vague feeling of discomfort in the upper abdomen, sometimes followed by borborygmi (rumbling or gurgling bowel sounds, and by a sensation of fullness in the head.

## Auranofin

A *gold* preparation used as an *antirheumatic drug* in the treatment of *rheumatoid arthritis*. Unlike other gold preparations, which are given as intramuscular injections, auranofin can be taken by mouth.

## Auricle

Another name for the pinna, the external flap of the *ear*. The term is also used to describe the earlike appendages of the atria (the upper chambers of the heart, see *atrium*).

## Auriscope

Also called an *otoscope*, an instrument for examining the ear.

## Auscultation

A procedure that involves listening to sounds within the body, using a *stethoscope*, to assess the functioning of an organ or to detect disease.

### AUSCULTATION OF THE HEART

To listen to the heart, the doctor places the stethoscope on the chest at four points which correspond to the location of the heart valves. With the patient either sitting up, lying in a semi-reclining position, or lying on his or her left side, the doctor listens for

# PROCEDURE FOR AUSCULTATION

A doctor's examination often includes auscultation (listening to sounds in the body using a stethoscope). Some sounds, such as movement of fluid through the stomach and intestine, opening and closing of heart valves, and flow of air through the lungs and airways, are made during normal functioning of organs. Abnormal sounds may indicate disease. An obstetrician listens for the baby's heartbeat as part of routine antenatal examination.

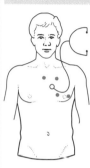

**The heart**
*The stethoscope is usually placed at four places on the chest overlying the sites of the heart valves. The doctor listens for the presence of murmurs, clicks, and extra heart sounds that may indicate disease of a heart valve.*

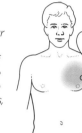

**The lungs**
*The doctor places the stethoscope over several different areas of the chest and back to listen to the sounds made during breathing. The presence of crackles and dry or moist wheezes indicates various types of lung disease.*

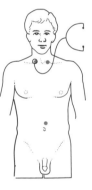

**Carotid artery and abdominal aorta**
*The doctor may listen to the flow of blood through blood vessels that pass just beneath the skin. The presence of bruits (sounds of turbulence) usually indicates abnormal narrowing or widening of an artery.*

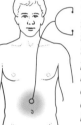

**The abdomen**
*The doctor may listen to the abdomen for the sounds made by the movement of fluid through the intestine. A disorder of the intestine may cause these sounds to be absent, abnormal, or very loud.*

## USING A STETHOSCOPE

The end is held against the skin. The diaphragm picks up most noises, while the bell detects quiet, deep noises.

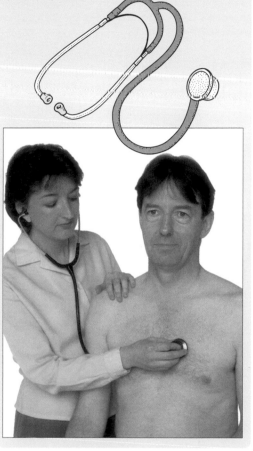

any abnormality in the rate and rhythm of the heartbeat and for a heart *murmur* or other abnormal *heart sound* that may indicate a heart defect.

## AUSCULTATION OF THE LUNGS

When listening to the lungs, the doctor places the stethoscope on numerous areas of the chest and back. The patient breathes normally, and then takes deep breaths, so that the doctor can compare the sounds on the right and left sides.

Abnormal breath sounds may indicate *pneumonia*, *bronchitis*, and *pneumothorax* (in which air enters the space between the *pleura*, the membranes lining the outside of the lungs and the inside of the chest cavity).

Cracking or bubbling sounds are caused by fluid in the lungs; wheezing sounds result from spasm of the airways, usually as a result of *asthma*.

*Pleurisy* (inflammation of the pleura) causes a scratching sound as inflamed areas of the lung rub together.

The doctor may also test for vocal resonance by asking the patient to whisper something.

The sound is louder if there is pus in the lung due to a condition such as pneumonia.

## AUSCULTATION OF BLOOD VESSELS

Blood vessels near the skin surface (the carotid artery in the neck, the abdominal aorta, or the renal artery) may be listened to for bruits (sounds made by turbulent or abnormally fast blood circulation). Bruits occur when blood vessels are narrowed by fatty deposits in *atherosclerosis* or widened (by an *aneurysm*, for example). They may also be present if heart valves have been narrowed or damaged (for example by *endocarditis*).

## AUSCULTATION OF THE ABDOMEN

The abdomen is auscultated for borborygmi (loud rumbling, gurgling

**A**

## AUTOGENIC TRAINING

Developed in Berlin in the 1920s, autogenic training (AT) claims to alleviate physical and mental problems, as well as improve work performance, creativity and personal relationships. It consists of a series of six mental exercises that allow the mind to calm itself by switching off the "fight-or-flight" stress responses of the body. The therapy offers a rational, organized way to relax at will and mobilize self-healing powers. A self-help treatment for stress-related conditions, AT became more established in the 1970s and is now practised worldwide.

### History

Autogenic training was developed in the 1920s by Dr. Johannes Schultz, a German neurologist and psychiatrist. "Autogenic" comes from the Greek for "generated from within". Dr. Schultz devised six silent verbal exercises for the mind which were further developed in Canada by his colleague, Dr. Wolfgang Luthe. Now available worldwide, it is used in some corporate staff-training programmes.

AT's therapeutic effects are reported in over 3,000 scientific papers, although these have not been validated. Physiological and brain-wave changes have been noted that, when measured, resemble those produced in meditation. The Schultz Institute in Berlin and the Oskar Vogt Institute in Japan are leading research centres.

### Consulting a practitioner

Autogenic training's structured approach has become relatively well established as a relaxation technique, and some doctors are beginning to refer patients for AT. It is usually taught in groups of six to eight patients, or on a one-to-one basis, in eight 90-minute weekly sessions.

Before tuition, you will be asked about your medical history, and interviewed for physical and psychological suitability. The six exercises taught by the practitioner are performed sitting or lying down, so comfortable clothes should be worn. Each exercise aims to induce relaxation in different areas of the body: heaviness in the neck, shoulders and limbs; warmth in the limbs; a calm heartbeat, relaxed

### Standard positions

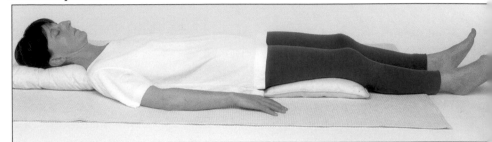

**Lying down** *is a useful position for practising autogenic exercises when going to sleep. Pillows are sometimes placed under the head and knees.*

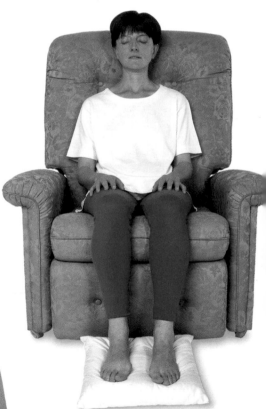

**Sitting in an upright chair** *is a position that can be used at work. It helps to relax the neck and shoulders, areas that often carry tension*

**Sitting in an armchair** *is a comfortable position, which can easily be adapted for practising AT in a bus, train or plane*

breathing, warmth in the stomach, and coolness in the forehead. Throughout the sequence, you will be asked to repeat set phrases, such as "my right arm is heavy", and, with practice, you should be able to reach an altered state of consciousness known as "passive concentration". This is similar to *meditation* and boosts the body's self-healing processes.

At a more advanced level, "autogenic modification" involves adopting formulas that focus on specific issues; someone with asthma, for example, may use the phrase "my sinuses are cool, my chest is warm".

Your practitioner can also teach you ways to cope with grief, anger, or anxiety, since repressed emotions ("autogenic discharges") may arise during treatment.

It is essential that you practise autogenic exercises between classes, for about 15 minutes, three times a day, noting your responses for the next session. Once taught, you can use the technique for self-treatment.

### Evidence and research

Autogenic training's therapeutic effects have been reported in over 3,000 scientific papers, although these have not been validated. Physiological and brain-wave changes have been noted that, when measured, resemble those produced in meditation. The Schultz Institute in Berlin and the Oskar Vogt Institute in Japan are leading research centres in this therapy.

### Medical opinion

Autogenic training's structured approach has become relatively well established and recognized as an effective relaxation technique, and some doctors may refer patients for AT.

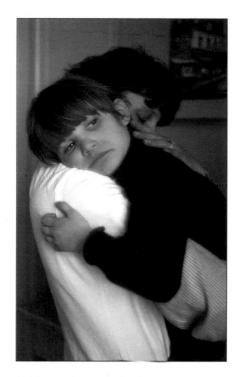

**Children with autism** *often have impaired communication and social skills, and they may exhibit unusual or difficult behaviour.*

sounds that are made by the movement of air and fluid in the intestine), and also for abnormal bowel sounds that may indicate intestinal obstruction (see *intestine, obstruction of*).

## Autism

A rare condition in which an affected person has difficulty with social relationships, communication, and with imagination, together with repetitive patterns of behaviour. Autism is more common in boys. The condition is, by definition, evident before the age of 30 months and is usually apparent in the first year of life. The precise causes of autism are unknown.

### SYMPTOMS AND SIGNS

Autistic children often seem normal for the first few months of life, before becoming increasingly unresponsive to parents or other stimuli. The child fails to form relationships, avoids eye contact, and has a preference for playing alone. Extreme resistance to change of any kind is an important feature of the condition, which can make it very difficult to teach the autistic child new skills.

Rituals develop in play, and there is often attachment to unusual objects or obsession with one particular idea. Delay in speaking is common and most autistic children have a low *IQ*.

Other behavioural abnormalities may include walking on tip-toe, rocking, self-injury, screaming fits, and *hyperactivity*

Appearance and coordination are normal. Some autistic people have an isolated special skill, such as musical ability or an outstanding rote memory.

### TREATMENT AND OUTLOOK

There is no cure for autism, which is a lifelong condition. Special schooling, support and *counselling* for the families, and, sometimes, *behaviour therapy* (such as to reduce violent self-injury) can be helpful. Medication is useful only for specific problems, such as hyperactivity.

The outlook depends on the intelligence and language ability of the individual. The majority of autistic people need special care.

## Autism spectrum disorders

A range of developmental disorders that are characterized by obsessive behaviour and impaired communication and social skills (see *Asperger's syndrome*; *autism*). Autism spectrum disorders are usually diagnosed during childhood.

## Autoantibody

An *antibody* (a protein that is manufactured by the immune system) that reacts against the body's own cells (see *autoimmune disorders*).

## Autogenic training

See box, left.

**A**

# Autoimmune disorders

Any of a number of disorders caused by a reaction of the body's *immune system* against its own cells and tissues. Such disease-producing processes, known as *hypersensitivity* reactions, are similar to the reactions that occur in *allergy*, except that in autoimmune disorders the hypersensitivity response is to the body itself rather than to an external substance.

## CAUSES
The immune system normally distinguishes "self" from "nonself". Some *lymphocytes* (a type of white blood cell) are capable of reacting against self, but these lymphocytes are generally suppressed. Autoimmune disorders occur when there is interruption of the normal control process, allowing such lymphocytes to escape from suppression, or when there is alteration in a particular body tissue meaning that it is no longer recognized as self and is attacked.

Bacteria, viruses, and drugs may play a role in initiating an autoimmune disorder in someone who already has a genetic (inherited) predisposition, but in most cases the trigger is unknown.

## TYPES
Autoimmune processes can have various results, such as the destruction of a particular type of cell or tissue, stimulation of an organ into excessive growth, or interference in an organ's function.

Autoimmune disorders are classified into organ-specific and non-organ-specific types. In organ-specific disorders, the autoimmune process is directed mainly against one organ. Examples include *Hashimoto's thyroiditis* (thyroid gland), pernicious *anaemia* (stomach), *Addison's disease* (adrenal glands), and type 1 *diabetes mellitus* (pancreas).

In non-organ-specific disorders, autoimmune activity is towards a tissue, such as connective tissue, that is widespread in the body. Examples of such disorders are systemic *lupus erythematosus* and *rheumatoid arthritis*.

## TREATMENT
Initial treatment for any autoimmune disorder is to reduce the effects of the disease by, for example, replacing hormones, such as insulin, that are not being produced.

In cases in which the disease is having widespread effects, treatment is also directed at diminishing the activity of the immune system while maintaining the body's ability to fight disease. *Corticosteroid drugs* are most commonly used for this purpose but may be combined with other *immunosuppressant drugs*.

# Autologous blood transfusion

See *blood transfusion, autologous*.

# Automatism

A state in which behaviour is not controlled by the conscious mind. An individual carries out activities without being aware of doing so, and later he or she has no clear memory of what happened. Episodes of automatism start abruptly and are usually no more than a few minutes in duration.

Automatism is uncommon and may be a symptom of *temporal lobe epilepsy*, *dissociative disorders* (psychological illnesses in which a particular mental function is lost), drug or *alcohol intoxication*, or *hypoglycaemia* (low blood sugar levels).

# Autonomic nervous system

Also called the involuntary nervous system, the part of the *nervous system* that controls the involuntary activities of a variety of body tissues, including blood vessels, organs, and glands. The autonomic nervous system consists of a network of nerves divided into the sympathetic and parasympathetic nervous systems.

The two systems act in conjunction and normally balance each other. However, during exercise or at times of stress, the activity of the sympathetic system predominates, while during sleep the parasympathetic system exerts greater control.

## SYMPATHETIC NERVOUS SYSTEM
The sympathetic nervous system comprises two chains of nerves that pass from the spinal cord throughout the body tissues. Into these tissues, the nerve endings release the *neurotransmitters* (chemical messengers) *adrenaline* (epinephrine) and *noradrenaline* (norepinephrine). The sympathetic nervous system also stimulates the release of adrenaline from the adrenal glands.

In general, the actions of the sympathetic nervous system heighten activity in the body. This activity is known as the *fight-or-flight response*. Among the most important effects produced are the acceleration and strengthening of the heartbeat, widening of the airways, widening of the blood vessels in muscles and narrowing of those in the skin and abdominal organs (in order to increase the blood flow through the muscles), and the inducement of sweating. In addition, the activity of the digestive system is decreased and the pupils are dilated.

## PARASYMPATHETIC NERVOUS SYSTEM
The parasympathetic nervous system is composed of a chain of nerves that passes from the brain and another that leaves the lower spinal cord. The nerves are distributed to the same tissues that are supplied by the sympathetic nerves. The parasympathetic nerves release

A

# YOUR BODY: FUNCTIONS OF THE AUTONOMIC NERVOUS SYSTEM

The autonomic nervous system (also known as the involuntary nervous system) is responsible for controlling the involuntary body functions, such as sweating, digestion, and heart rate. The system affects smooth muscles, such as those of the airways and the intestine, rather than the striated muscles, which are under the body's voluntary control.

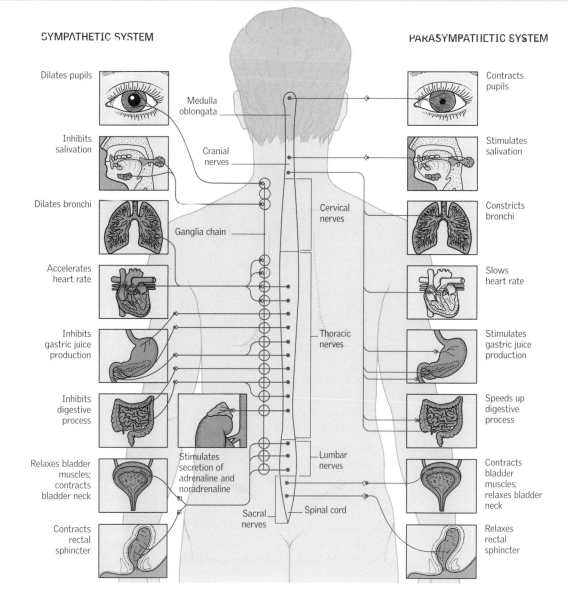

**SYMPATHETIC SYSTEM**

Dilates pupils

Inhibits salivation

Dilates bronchi

Accelerates heart rate

Inhibits gastric juice production

Inhibits digestive process

Relaxes bladder muscles; contracts bladder neck

Contracts rectal sphincter

Medulla oblongata

Cranial nerves

Ganglia chain

Cervical nerves

Thoracic nerves

Stimulates secretion of adrenaline and noradrenaline

Lumbar nerves

Sacral nerves

Spinal cord

**PARASYMPATHETIC SYSTEM**

Contracts pupils

Stimulates salivation

Constricts bronchi

Slows heart rate

Stimulates gastric juice production

Speeds up digestive process

Contracts bladder muscles; relaxes bladder neck

Relaxes rectal sphincter

### The autonomic nervous system

*The autonomic nervous system is divided into two separate systems: the sympathetic nervous system and the parasympathetic nervous system. The sympathetic system is primarily concerned with preparing the body for action; it predominates at times of stress or excitement. The sympathetic system stimulates functions such as heart-rate and sweating and dilates the blood vessels to the muscles so that more blood is diverted to them. Simultaneously, it subdues the activity of the digestive system. In contrast, the parasympathetic nervous system is concerned mainly with the body's everyday functions such as digestion and the excretion of waste products; this system dominates during sleep. The parasympathetic system slows the heart rate and stimulates the organs of the digestive tract. Most of the time, activity is balanced between the two systems, with neither dominating. Both of the systems play an important part in sexual arousal and orgasm.*

## YOUR BODY: CHROMOSOMES AND AUTOSOMES

Present in all nucleated body cells, chromosomes are thread-like structures that carry the genetic code for the body. The nucleus of a human cell contains 46 chromosomes, each of which is a long, coiled molecule of DNA, and together they contain about 35,000 genes. Every gene is a tiny segment of DNA that controls a particular cell function by governing the synthesis (manufacture) of a specific protein. The chromosomes are matched up and arranged into the 22 pairs of autosomes and one pair of sex chromosomes. A study of the complete set will reveal any abnormalities.

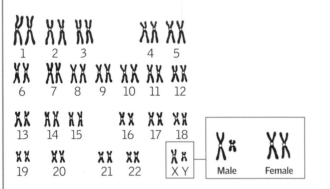

**Human genetic inheritance**
*Human genes are arranged on 22 pairs of matching chromosomes – also known as autosomes – plus two sex chromosomes. One chromosome in each pair is inherited from each parent.*

**Chromosome**
*Each chromosome consists of a long, tightly coiled molecule of DNA.*

the neurotransmitter acetylcholine, which has the opposite effect to those of adrenaline and noradrenaline. The parasympathetic system is concerned mainly with everyday functions such as digestion and excretion.

### EFFECT OF DRUGS
Certain disorders can be treated with drugs that affect the autonomic nervous system. *Anticholinergic drugs*, for example, block the effect of acetylcholine, which can reduce muscle spasms in the intestine. *Beta-blocker drugs* block the action of adrenaline and noradrenaline on the heart, thus slowing the rate and force of the heartbeat. (See box, previous page.)

## Autopsy

A postmortem examination of the body, including the internal organs, which is usually undertaken to determine the cause of death. An autopsy is sometimes required by law.

When the cause of death is known and there are no legal requirements for an autopsy to be carried out, hospitals and/or doctors may seek the next-of-kin's permission to perform an autopsy in order to advance knowledge of the disease that caused death, thereby helping in the care of future patients with the same condition. Relatives are free to refuse such consent.

## Autoregulation

Processes occurring within the body that maintain ideal conditions for normal function. Such processes include the distribution of blood between different organs, and balance of the body's salt and water content.

## Autosomal disorders

See *genetic disorders*.

## Autosome

Any *chromosome* (see box left) that is not a sex chromosome. Of the 23 pairs of chromosomes in each human cell, 22 pairs are autosomes. (See box left.)

## Autosuggestion

This term refers to putting oneself into a receptive hypnotic-like state as a means of stimulating the body's ability to heal itself. The idea that symptoms could be relieved merely through attitude was put forward by the Frenchman Emile Coué at the end of the nineteenth century.

Although, autosuggestion enjoyed only brief popularity, some techniques that are used today are based on its premise. For example, in one method used to control anxiety symptoms, people are taught muscular relaxation techniques (see *biofeedback*) and learn to summon up calming imagery or pleasant thoughts.

## Avascular

A term meaning without blood vessels.

## Avascular necrosis

Cell death in body tissues as a result of damage to the blood vessels that supply the area.

## Aversion therapy

An outdated form of *behaviour therapy* in which unpleasant stimuli, such as electric shocks, are administered at the same time as an unwanted behaviour is exhibited in an attempt to alter such behavioural patterns. Other forms of therapy are now generally considered to be more appropriate.

# Aviation medicine

The medical speciality concerned with the physiological effects of air travel, such as the effects of reduced oxygen, pressure changes, and accelerative forces, as well as with the causes and treatment of medical problems that may occur during a flight.

Aviation medicine includes assessment of the fitness of the aircrew, and sometimes of passengers, to fly, the management of medical emergencies in the air, the consequences of special types of flights (such as in helicopters and spacecraft), and the investigation of aircraft accidents.

AIR-TRAVEL-RELATED PROBLEMS
Increasing altitude causes a fall in air pressure and with it a fall in the pressure of oxygen. *Hypoxia* (a seriously reduced oxygen concentration in the blood and tissues) is a threat to anyone who flies at altitude. Aviator's *decompression sickness* has the same causes as the related condition that affects scuba divers but it is not normally a risk for passengers on regular flights. Rapid decompression (a sudden drop in air pressure) in civil aircraft is extremely rare, but passengers and crew are provided with oxygen masks for use in emergencies while the aircraft descends to a safe altitude.

Hypoxia or, more commonly, anxiety during flight can lead to *hyper-ventilation* (overbreathing), in which increased breathing results in excess loss of carbon dioxide. This loss alters the body's acidity and gives rise to symptoms such as tingling around the mouth, muscle spasms, and lightheadedness. If such symptoms develop, the treatment is to rebreathe air from a paper bag held over the nose and mouth, which reduces the loss of carbon dioxide.

The changes in altitude or cabin pressure during a flight affect the body's gas-containing cavities, principally the middle ears, the facial

sinuses, the lungs, and the intestines. When pressure drops during ascent, the volume of gas in these cavities increases and usually escapes freely. On descent, the gas volume decreases as pressure outside the body rises. Unless preventative measures are taken, this may cause pain and, rarely, damage (see *barotrauma*). There is increasing concern about the risk of

developing deep vein thrombosis (see *thrombosis, deep vein*) during air travel. The condition may be caused by long periods of sitting in one position or compression of the tissues, both of which occur during long-haul flights.

The accelerative forces experienced by passengers travelling in civil aircraft are mild, even during take-off and landing, and no medical

## CONDITIONS AFFECTING PASSENGER SUITABILITY FOR AIR TRAVEL

Pressure changes, accelerative forces, and reduced oxygen levels, all have an effect on the body during air travel. Due to these physiological effects, there are certain medical conditions and ailments that could be cause for concern, such as a recent stroke or severe anaemia. If you are affected by any of the conditions listed below, seek the advice of your doctor before flying.

| Conditions | Comments |
| --- | --- |
| Lung disease (such as chronic bronchitis or emphysema)<br><br>Severe anaemia<br><br>Heart condition (such as angina pectoris, heart failure, or recent heart attack) | The lowered cabin pressure (and thus the oxygen level) at higher altitudes aggravates an already impaired ability to oxygenate the blood and/or tissues and may cause severe respiratory distress or collapse. Seek your doctor's advice. Flying may be possible if you are able to walk 50 metres without breathlessness or chest pain. |
| Recent stroke | Seek your doctor's advice. You may need to wait some weeks before flying. |
| Recent surgery to inner or middle ear, abdomen, chest, or brain; a recently collapsed lung or a fractured skull. | Seek your doctor's advice. You may need to wait before flying to avoid damage to your hearing mechanism from the expansion of gas trapped in the chest, abdomen, or skull. |
| Pregnancy | No flying after 34 to 36 weeks on most airlines. |
| Newborn baby | An infant should not fly until at least 48 hours old. |
| Psychiatric disorder | May need trained escort. |
| Infectious disease, terminal illness, or vomiting | May be refused entry to aircraft: Check with airline. |

**A**

## YOUR BODY: THE MOVEMENT OF THE AXIS

Joints are formed where two or more bones meet. Most joints, including those of the limbs, move freely and are known as synovial joints. They are lubricated by synovial fluid secreted by the joint lining. There are different types of synovial joint, including ball-and-socket, hinge, and ellipsoidal. In a pivot joint, one bone rotates within a collar formed by another. The pivot joint between the atlas and the axis, the uppermost bones of the neck, allows the head to turn to either side.

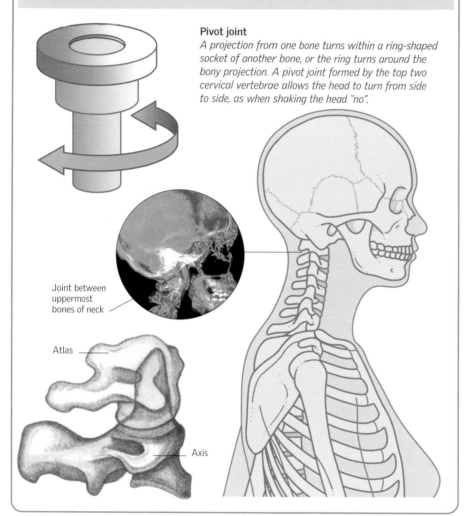

**Pivot joint**
*A projection from one bone turns within a ring-shaped socket of another bone, or the ring turns around the bony projection. A pivot joint formed by the top two cervical vertebrae allows the head to turn from side to side, as when shaking the head "no".*

Joint between uppermost bones of neck

Atlas

Axis

precautions are necessary. Military aircraft pilots, on the other hand, may experience severe accelerations and must wear special suits and use a reclined seat to prevent pooling of blood in the feet, which would cause immediate loss of consciousness.

*Motion sickness* usually causes fewer problems during air travel than during road or sea travel. Passengers who are prone to motion sickness may benefit from taking an anti-motion sickness preparation.

Air travel often involves the rapid crossing of several time zones within a short period of time, which can affect sleep-waking cycles, causing jet-lag.

AVIATION MEDICINE SPECIALISTS
Most large airlines have doctors who are specially trained in aviation medicine who are responsible for the healthcare of the airline staff. The doctors also give advice on the transportation of sick passengers, the provision of training and any equipment required to deal with illness during flight, and the maintenance of airline hygiene. (See box, previous page.)

## Avulsed tooth

A tooth that has become completely dislodged from its socket following an injury. If the tooth is kept clean and moist (ideally by being stored in milk, saliva, or contact-lens solution), is not otherwise washed, and treatment is sought immediately, reimplantation (see *reimplantation, dental*) may be possible.

## Avulsion

The tearing away of a body structure from its point of attachment. Avulsion may be due to an injury, for example excessive contraction of a *tendon* may avulse a small piece of bone at its attachment point. Avulsion may also be performed as part of a surgical procedure, as in the surgical removal of *varicose veins*.

## Axilla

The medical name for the armpit.

## Axis

The second cervical *vertebra* in the *spine*. The axis is attached by a pivot joint to the *atlas*, the top vertebra, which is attached to the base of the skull. The pivot joint allows the head to turn to either side. (See box, left)

## Axon

The thin, elongated part of a *neuron* (nerve cell) that conducts nerve impulses. Many axons in the body are covered with a fatty myelin sheath. (See box, below right.)

A

## Ayurvedic medicine

See box overleaf.

## Azathioprine

An *immunosuppressant drug* used to treat severe *rheumatoid arthritis* and other *autoimmune disorders* (in which the *immune system* attacks the body's own tissues). It is also used to prevent organ rejection after *transplant surgery*. Azathioprine may be injected or given in tablet form. Side effects include increased susceptibility to infection.

## Azelaic acid

A *topical* (applied to the skin) drug used to treat mild to moderate *acne*.

## Azithromycin

A macrolide *antibiotic drug* used to treat infections of the skin, chest, throat, and ears. Azithromycin is also used to treat genital infections due to chlamydia (see *chlamydial infections*).

## Azoospermia

The absence of sperm from semen, causing *infertility* in males. Azoospermia may be caused either by a *congenital* disorder or by one that develops later in life. It can also occur following a *vasectomy*.

### CAUSES
Congenital azoospermia may be due to a *chromosomal abnormality* such as *Klinefelter's syndrome* (the presence of an extra sex chromosome); failure of the testes to descend into the scrotum; absence of the vasa deferentia (the ducts that carry sperm from the testes to the seminal vesicles, where it is stored prior to ejaculation); or *cystic fibrosis* (a genetic disease of the lungs and pancreas that may also cause defects of the vasa deferentia).

In some males, azoospermia may be the result of hormonal disorders affecting the onset of puberty. Another cause is blockage of the vasa deferentia, which may follow a *sexually transmitted infection*, *tuberculosis*, or surgery on the groin.

Azoospermia can also be the result of damage to the testes. This can follow *radiotherapy*, treatment with certain drugs (for example, *anticancer drugs*), prolonged exposure to heat, or the effects of occupational exposure to toxic chemicals. In some cases, production of sperm ceases permanently for no known reason.

### TREATMENT AND OUTLOOK
If the cause is treatable (with hormones to bring on puberty or surgery to unblock ducts closed by infection, for example), sperm production may restart. However, in some cases the testes will have been permanently damaged.

## AZT

The abbreviation for azidothymidine, the former name for *zidovudine*.

## Aztreonam

An *antibiotic drug* used to treat some types of *meningitis* and infections by certain types of bacteria, including *Pseudomonas*.

## Azygous

A term meaning not paired. Azygous describes a structure such as the heart, which does not have a twin organ on the opposite side of the body (as opposed to the kidney, which does have a twin organ). The azygous vein drains blood from the abdomen and chest and travels along the right side of the spine.

---

### YOUR BODY: AXON

The basic unit of the nervous system is a special cell called a neuron, or nerve cell. This has a cell body with a central nucleus and various other structures that are important for maintaining cell life. Neurons have long projections, or processes, known as axons (nerve fibres) and dendrites. Axons carry nerve impulses away from the cell; dendrites receive impulses from other neurons.

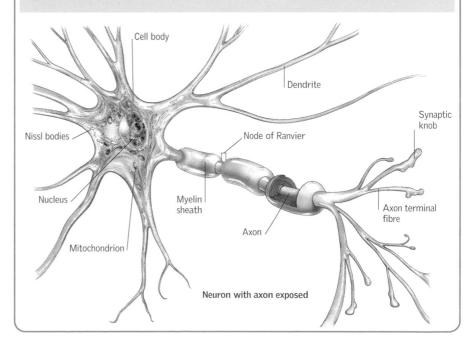

Cell body
Dendrite
Synaptic knob
Nissl bodies
Node of Ranvier
Nucleus
Myelin sheath
Axon terminal fibre
Mitochondrion
Axon

**Neuron with axon exposed**

# AYURVEDA

The major traditional holistic healing system of the Indian subcontinent, Ayurveda covers all aspects of health, encouraging physical, mental, emotional, and spiritual well-being. Practitioners believe that well-being is affected by three *doshas*, or "vital energies", which constantly fluctuate. Treatment aims to restore health, or *doshic* balance, through purifying techniques, diet, yoga postures and breathing exercises, massage, and herbal remedies. Ayurveda is currently undergoing a government-sponsored revival in India, and is attracting much interest in the West, particularly in the United States.

### History
Ayurveda (Sanskrit for "science of life") has been used on the Indian subcontinent since about 2500 BC. Derived from the *Vedas*, ancient Hindu texts by *rishis*, or holy men, it is a sophisticated, comprehensive health system, and has similarities with Traditional Chinese Medicine.

For thousands of years, Ayurveda was a well-regulated oral tradition. It remained the most accessible form of healthcare for Indians until the 19th century, when the British Raj attempted to stamp it out, resulting in a proliferation of poorly trained practitioners. Following Indian independence in 1947, Ayurveda began a revival.

### Key principles
Ayurveda teaches that there are five great elements – ether, air, fire, water, and earth – which underlie all living systems and are constantly changing and interacting. They can be simplified into three *doshas*, or vital energies, existing in ever-changing proportions throughout nature.

In the human body, the levels of the *doshas* are believed to rise and fall daily, affected by factors such as different foods, time of day, season, levels of stress and repressed emotions. Imbalances in the *doshas* are thought to disrupt the flow of *prana*, the "life energy" that enters the body through food and breath, and to impede *agni*, the body's "digestive fire", which processes food and experiences. If *agni* is low, toxic substances called *ama* are produced, said to be a major source of illness.

Ayurveda therefore places great importance on diet and detoxification techniques designed to purge *ama* by means of sweat, urine, and faeces – known as the three *malas*. Herbal remedies, yoga, massage, and meditation are also believed to balance the *doshas* and increase *prana*, and are all practised as part of Ayurveda.

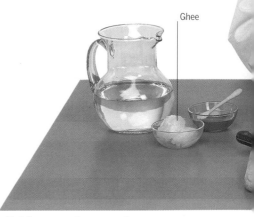

The practitioner *mixes a remedy to suit the patient's individual type. An Ayurvedic prescription is likely to include at least ten different herbs.*

Ghee

### Evidence and research
Much research into Ayurvedic medicine has been carried out in India. Many Western doctors accept that they cannot discount the medical systems of other

## STANDARD TESTS

The practitioner may listen to your internal organs and use other diagnostic techniques shown here.

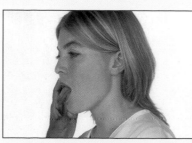

**The tongue** *is examined for signs of toxins in the body.*

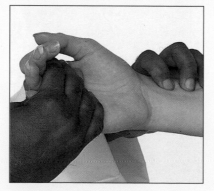

**The pulse** *is taken to reveal the* doshic *state of related body organs.*

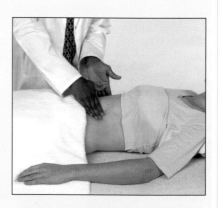

**Palpating or feeling the abdomen** *may reveal* doshic *imbalances.*

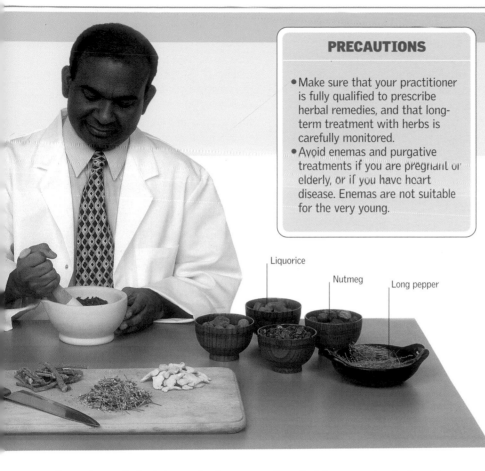

Liquorice

Nutmeg

Long pepper

## PRECAUTIONS

- Make sure that your practitioner is fully qualified to prescribe herbal remedies, and that long-term treatment with herbs is carefully monitored.
- Avoid enemas and purgative treatments if you are pregnant or elderly, or if you have heart disease. Enemas are not suitable for the very young.

## ASSESSING THE STATE OF THE *DOSHAS*

The patient's physical appearance and the way she moves are closely examined as aids to diagnosis. The eyes and nails can be important indications of *doshic* constitution. *Pitta* types, for example, tend to have bright, sparkling eyes.

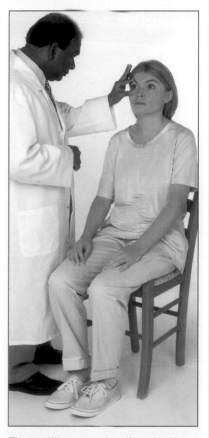

*The practitioner examines the patient's eyes for clues to her balance of* doshas.

cultures. Ayurvedic herbal remedies have been tried and tested by centuries of use, but their quality and efficacy cannot be guaranteed, since very few scientific tests have been done. Doctors find Ayurveda's emphasis on health promotion, and its belief that illness is caused by factors such as diet and lifestyle, easier to accept than some of its treatments. Most would consider that anyone with a critical illness is better off with conventional medicine.

### Consulting a practitioner

At the first consultation, the practitioner identifies your *doshic* constitution (*tridosha*) and any imbalances in it. He asks detailed questions about your personal and family history and about your lifestyle, from eating and bowel habits to relationships at work. As in Traditional Chinese Medicine, taking the pulse is an important part of diagnosis. The practitioner checks the pulse at three points on both wrists, each thought to correspond to one of the *doshas* and to reflect the condition of specific internal organs. You may also

be asked for a sample of urine, taken in midstream early in the morning; its colour and odour will be noted.

Your practitioner will recommend dietary changes to rebalance your *doshas*. He will advise you to eat at certain times of day, depending on your age and condition, your *doshic* type, and the season of the year. If qualified to give medicinal remedies, your practitioner will also prescribe herbs or minerals according to your constitution and *doshic* imbalance. This is part of a programme known as *shaman*, which aims to pacify and calm the *doshas*.

If the practitioner considers you strong enough, he may begin with a cleansing and detoxifying regime called *shodan*, which takes the form of enemas, laxatives, therapeutic vomiting and washing out the nasal passages, collectively known as "*panchakarma*". This means "five actions" and is a unification process to remove *ama*, or impurities, in the body, and to rebalance the *doshas*. It requires physical strength, and should always be carefully monitored by a trained practitioner.

Traditionally, *panchakarma* is performed in three stages after a restricted diet or fast. Massage with medicated oils is followed by induced sweating, which is said to return the *doshas* to their seats in the body. The main purging process is achieved with herbal or oil enemas, herbal laxatives or induced vomiting.

Finally, the practitioner may suggest *rasayana*, a rejuvenating regime that may include herbal remedies, yoga, chanting, meditation (*satvajaya*), and sunbathing.

# Babesiosis

A general term covering a number of diseases that are caused by the *BABESIA* genus of *protozoa* (single-celled *parasites*.)

Babesiosis is mainly a disease of animals; it may affect sheep, cattle, horses, and other domestic animals. Babesiosis can be transmitted from animals to humans by tick bites, producing symptoms similar to those of *malaria*.

Treatment is with the antimalarial drug *quinine* and an *antibiotic drug*. (See also *ticks and disease*.)

# Babinski's sign

A *reflex* movement in which the big toe bends upwards when the outer edge of the sole of the foot is scratched. In babies, Babinski's sign is a normal reflex action. In adults, Babinski's sign is an indication of damage to, or disease of, the *brain* or the *spinal cord*.

# Bach flower remedies

See box, opposite.

# Bacillary dysentery

A type of *dysentery* (infection of the intestinal tract) caused by bacteria of the *SHIGELLA* genus (see *shigellosis*).

# *Bacille Calmette-Guérin*

See *BCG vaccination*.

# Bacilli

Rod-shaped *bacteria*. Bacilli (singular: bacillus) are responsible for causing a variety of diseases, including *infectious diseases* such as tuberculosis, tetanus, typhoid fever, pertussis (whooping cough), and diphtheria.

# Bacitracin

A type of *antibiotic drug* used in combination with other drugs to treat infections of the eyes and skin. Bacitracin is most commonly applied as an external skin preparation or as eye-drops.

# Back

The area between the shoulders and buttocks. The back is supported by the spinal column (see *spine*), which is bound together by *ligaments* (bands of tough, fibrous tissue) and supported by muscles that also help to control posture and movement.

## DISORDERS

Back problems are numerous and may be the result of a variety of factors affecting the spine. They can be related to disorders of bones, muscles, ligaments, tendons, nerves, and joints in the spine, all of which can cause back pain. (See also *spine* disorders box.)

# Background radiation

The small amounts of natural *radiation* that emanate from such sources as rocks and the soil.

# Back pain

Most people suffer from back pain at some time in their lives. In many cases, no exact diagnosis is made because the pain gets better with rest and because analgesic drugs (painkillers) are used before any tests, such as X-rays, are carried out. In such cases, doctors may use the term "nonspecific back pain" to describe the condition.

## CAUSES

Nonspecific back pain is one of the largest single causes of working days lost through illness in the UK. The people most likely to suffer from back pain are those whose jobs involve a lot of heavy lifting and carrying or those who spend long periods sitting in one position or bending awkwardly. Overweight people are also more prone to back pain – their backs carry a heavier load and they tend to have weaker abdominal muscles, which usually help to provide support to the back.

Nonspecific back pain is thought to be caused by a mechanical disorder affecting one or more structures in the back. This may be a ligament strain, a muscle tear, damage to a spinal facet joint, or *disc prolapse* (slipped disc).

In addition to pain from a damaged structure, spasm of surrounding muscles will cause pain and tenderness over a wider area. This can result in temporary *scoliosis* (an abnormal sideways curvature of the spine).

Abnormalities of a facet joint and prolapse of an intervertebral disc can both cause *sciatica* (pain in the buttock and down the back of the leg into the foot). This condition is the result of pressure on a sciatic nerve root as it leaves the spinal cord. Coughing, sneezing, or straining will increase the pain. Pressure on the sciatic nerve can also cause a *pins-and-needles* sensation in that leg as well as weakness in muscles that are activated by the nerve. Rarely, pain may radiate down the femoral nerve at the front of the thigh.

Osteoarthritis in the joints of the spine can cause persistent back pain. *Ankylosing spondylitis* (an inflammatory disorder in which arthritis affects the spine) causes back pain and stiffness with loss of back mobility. *Coccydynia* (pain and tenderness at the base of the spine) may occur after a fall in which the coccyx has struck the ground, during pregnancy, or spontaneously for unknown reasons.

Fibrositis is an imprecise term that is sometimes used to describe pain and tenderness in muscles, which may

**continued on page 166**

# BACH FLOWER REMEDIES

Dr. Edward Bach was an English doctor who concluded from studies of his patients that negative emotions could lead to physical illness. He was also convinced that flowers possessed healing properties that could be used to treat emotional problems and so restore health and harmony to mind and body. In the 1930s, Dr. Bach began to produce his remedies, which are made by infusing or boiling plant material in spring water.

Gorse

## Main uses

Bach Flower Remedies and other flower essences are today popular around the world, and are often taken for self-help during times of emotional crisis or stress. The main uses are negative emotional states, such as fearfulness, uncertainty, disinterest, loneliness, over-sensitivity, despair and excessive concern for others, and any physical symptoms arising from emotional problems.

## History

Early in the 20th century, a London doctor and homeopath, Dr. Edward Bach (pronounced "batch") made a study of his patients and concluded that harmful emotions, such as despair or fearfulness, could lead to physical disease. Convinced that flowers could affect one's state of mind, and familiar with the homeopathic law of potentization, Dr. Bach developed his Flower Remedies. He identified these by holding his hand over each flower in the belief that he could intuitively discern its healing properties. By 1936, Bach's remedies were being made commercially. They are now available from natural-health outlets worldwide.

Oak

## Consulting a practitioner

Although practitioners in other fields, such as homeopathy, naturopathy, and aromatherapy, may sometimes prescribe Bach Flower Remedies, Dr. Bach developed his remedies primarily for self-help use. Several remedies may be taken together, and the selection is generally based on the patient's assessment of his or her emotional state. However, some people select the individual remedies by holding a pendulum over each in turn.

Bach remedies are not intended directly to relieve the physical symptoms of an ailment. Dr. Bach believed that harmful emotions were the main cause of disease, and he sought to treat moods such as fear, anger, guilt and depression in order to restore the harmony of mind and body that he believed to be necessary for good health.

Dr. Bach classified the various moods into seven emotional groups, which he then subdivided into 38 negative feelings, each one associated with a particular plant. He also developed a special compound, called Rescue Remedy, to be taken for shock, panic and hysteria.

Remedies are prepared by infusion, with flower heads placed on the surface of pure spring water and left to infuse in direct sunlight for three hours; or by boiling short lengths of twigs with flowers or catkins in pure spring water for 30 minutes. After either process, the water is retained and preserved in brandy.

Bach remedies are sold in a concentrated form, which should be diluted in fruit juice or mineral water, rubbed on the lips or behind the ears, or dropped directly on the tongue. The dose is usually four drops of solution, repeated four times a day. For immediate problems, the dose may be repeated every 3–5 minutes until symptoms subside.

## Evidence and research

No clinical trials have been carried out on Bach Flower Remedies, and in chemical analysis only spring water and alcohol were detected. One theory attributes any effects to a kind of "molecular imprinting", but this idea is controversial and claims of efficacy are anecdotal.

The unorthodox methods by which Dr. Bach identified and produced his remedies, together with stories of patients choosing their own remedies by dowsing, have, not surprisingly, left most doctors unimpressed by the claims made for Bach Flower Remedies. Doctors are likely to attribute any benefits derived from them to the placebo response.

*Bach Flower Remedies are sold in 10 ml and 20 ml "stock" phials, containing individual remedies in a concentrated solution. They should always be stored in a cool, dark place.*

10 ml phial

20 ml phial

Crab apple

Honeysuckle

Heather

## SELF HELP: PREVENTING BACK PAIN

Most people have experienced back pain at some time in their lives, but in many cases the problem could have been avoided. Back pain may be due to poor posture, weak abdominal or back muscles, or sudden muscle strain. You can improve your posture by wearing comfortable shoes, by standing or sitting with your spine properly aligned, and by choosing an appropriate mattress for your bed. Regular exercises strengthen abdominal and back muscles, and losing excess weight will relieve stress on joints and muscles. Learning how to perform physical tasks safely, including how to lift and carry objects, can help to prevent back strain. Ask your doctor or physiotherapist to give you advice on posture, exercises, and diet.

### Correct body posture

To break bad postural habits, you should be constantly aware of the way in which you stand, sit, move, and even sleep. The pictures on this page show how to carry out everyday activities comfortably, with minimal strain on your spine and back muscles.

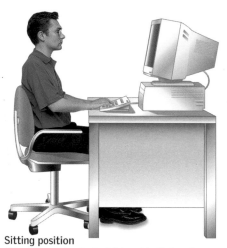

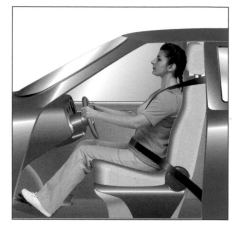

Shoulders pulled back

Trunk held straight

Abdominal muscles tightened

Pelvis tilted slightly to align body

**B**

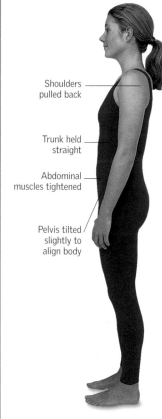

#### Sitting position
*Sit with your back straight and both feet flat on the floor. Use a chair that supports the small of your back. When using a computer, position the monitor so that you can look straight at it.*

#### Driving position
*Before setting off, angle the back of your seat so that it supports your spine, and position the seat so that you can reach the hand and foot controls comfortably, without straining.*

### Back-strengthening exercises

You can help to prevent back pain by gently exercising the muscles in your back and abdomen. See a doctor or ask for a referral to a physiotherapist before starting a programme of exercise. You should not continue to do any exercise that causes you pain. The movements shown below should make your back muscles stronger and your spine more flexible. Repeat each one 10 times if you can, and try to exercise daily. Do the exercises on a comfortable but firm, flat surface, such as a mat laid on the floor.

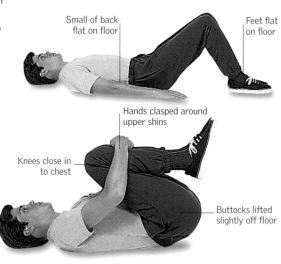

Small of back flat on floor

Feet flat on floor

Hands clasped around upper shins

Knees close in to chest

Buttocks lifted slightly off floor

### Standing position
*Put your weight evenly on both feet. Hold your head up and shoulders back, allowing your spine to curve naturally. Balance your body over its centre of gravity, which is in the pelvis and lower spine.*

### Lower back stretch
*This stretch may relieve aching joints and muscles in the lower back. Lie on your back with your feet flat on the floor and with your knees bent. Lift your knees towards your body. With your hands, pull your knees into your chest. Hold for 7 seconds and breathe deeply. Keeping your knees bent, lower your feet to the floor one at a time.*

## LIFTING A HEAVY OBJECT

When lifting, pushing, or pulling a heavy object, keep the object close to you so that you can use your full strength to move it. To lift an object, hold the bottom edge so that you support the full weight of the object and keep your body balanced as you lift to avoid straining your spine.

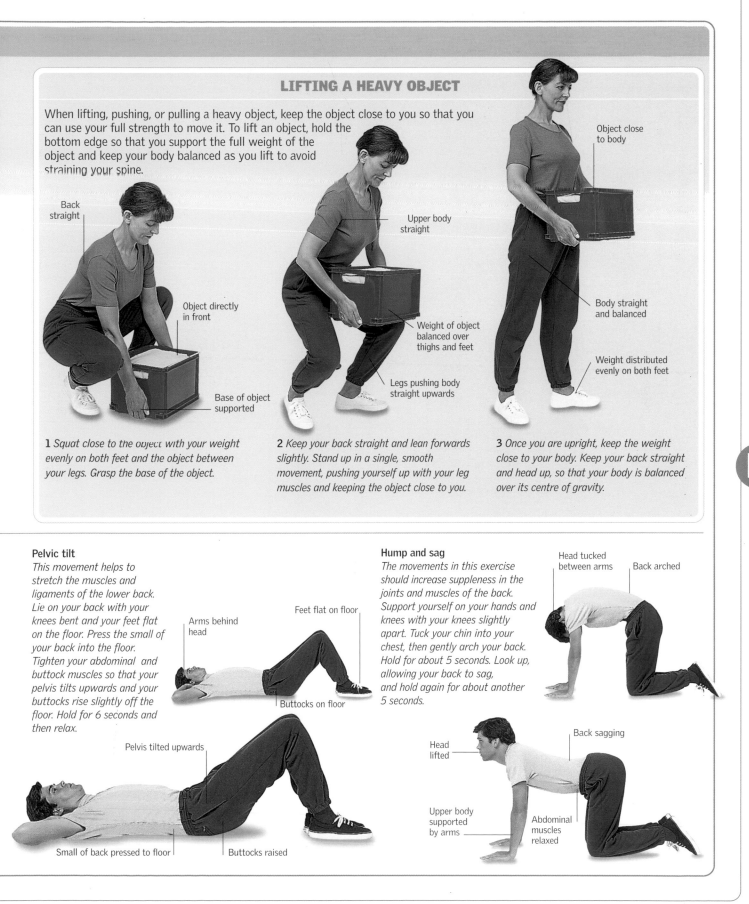

Object close to body

Back straight

Object directly in front

Base of object supported

Upper body straight

Weight of object balanced over thighs and feet

Legs pushing body straight upwards

Body straight and balanced

Weight distributed evenly on both feet

**1** *Squat close to the object with your weight evenly on both feet and the object between your legs. Grasp the base of the object.*

**2** *Keep your back straight and lean forwards slightly. Stand up in a single, smooth movement, pushing yourself up with your leg muscles and keeping the object close to you.*

**3** *Once you are upright, keep the weight close to your body. Keep your back straight and head up, so that your body is balanced over its centre of gravity.*

**B**

### Pelvic tilt

*This movement helps to stretch the muscles and ligaments of the lower back. Lie on your back with your knees bent and your feet flat on the floor. Press the small of your back into the floor. Tighten your abdominal and buttock muscles so that your pelvis tilts upwards and your buttocks rise slightly off the floor. Hold for 6 seconds and then relax.*

Arms behind head

Feet flat on floor

Buttocks on floor

Pelvis tilted upwards

Small of back pressed to floor

Buttocks raised

### Hump and sag

*The movements in this exercise should increase suppleness in the joints and muscles of the back. Support yourself on your hands and knees with your knees slightly apart. Tuck your chin into your chest, then gently arch your back. Hold for about 5 seconds. Look up, allowing your back to sag, and hold again for about another 5 seconds.*

Head tucked between arms

Back arched

Head lifted

Back sagging

Upper body supported by arms

Abdominal muscles relaxed

## BACK PAIN

Most people experience back pain at some time in their lives, but in most cases it is not serious and the problem corrects itself before investigation takes place. However, some kinds of back pain can be related to a specific disorder. The most common sites affected by back pain are shown here.

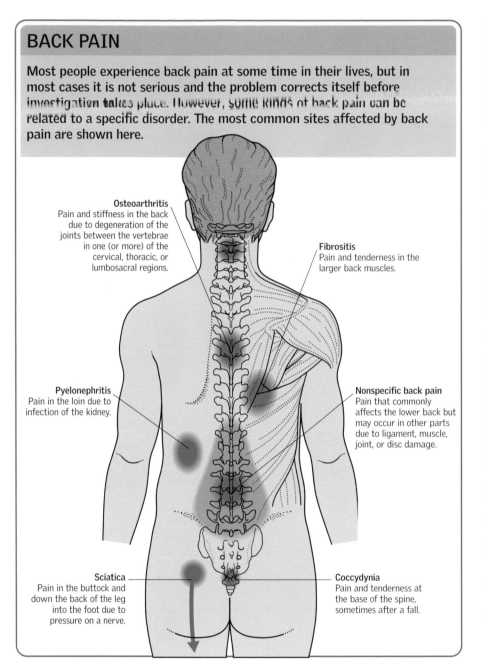

**Osteoarthritis**
Pain and stiffness in the back due to degeneration of the joints between the vertebrae in one (or more) of the cervical, thoracic, or lumbosacral regions.

**Fibrositis**
Pain and tenderness in the larger back muscles.

**Pyelonephritis**
Pain in the loin due to infection of the kidney.

**Nonspecific back pain**
Pain that commonly affects the lower back but may occur in other parts due to ligament, muscle, joint, or disc damage.

**Sciatica**
Pain in the buttock and down the back of the leg into the foot due to pressure on a nerve.

**Coccydynia**
Pain and tenderness at the base of the spine, sometimes after a fall.

affect the back. Fibrositis is often worse in cold and damp weather and is occasionally associated with feeling generally unwell. Unlike other causes of back pain, fibrositis is not accompanied by muscle spasm or restriction of back movement. It often improves when treated with non-steroidal anti-inflammatory drugs.

*Pyelonephritis* can cause back pain as well as pain and tenderness in the loin, fever, chills, and pain on passing urine. Cancer in the spine can cause

persistent back pain that disturbs sleep and is not relieved by rest.

### SELF-HELP
People with back pain and sciatica are usually advised to remain as mobile as possible. Sleeping on a firm mattress and taking analgesic drugs can help to relieve pain. However, if pain persists, is very severe, or is associated with weakness in a leg or bladder control problems, immediate medical advice should be sought.

### INVESTIGATION
Examination of the back may show tenderness in specific areas or loss of back mobility. Weakness or loss of sensation in the legs implies pressure on a nerve root, which needs prompt investigation.

X-rays of the spine may reveal narrowing between the intervertebral discs; osteoarthritis; *osteoporosis;* ankylosing spondylitis; compression fracture; stress fracture; *bone cancer;* or *spondylolisthesis* (displacement of vertebrae). X-rays will not reveal ligament, muscle, facet joint, or disc damage. To detect pressure on a nerve root (due to disc prolapse, for example), *myelography, CT scanning,* or *MRI* is performed.

### TREATMENT
If a specific cause is found for the back pain, treatment will be for that cause. Research has shown that acute nonspecific back pain is best treated by early return to normal activity, helped by analgesic drugs. Bed rest should not be continued for more than two days. Chronic nonspecific back pain is often more difficult to treat. Treatment may include use of *aspirin* and related drugs, *nonsteroidal anti-inflammatory drugs, muscle-relaxant drugs, acupuncture,* or spinal injection. Exercise, spinal *manipulation,* or wearing a surgical *corset* may also be helpful; and spinal surgery may sometimes be necessary. (See also box left and previous page.)

# Baclofen

A *muscle-relaxant drug* that blocks nerve activity in the spinal cord. Baclofen is used to relieve muscle *spasm* and stiffness caused by injury to either the brain or spinal cord, by neurological disorders such as *multiple sclerosis,* or by a *stroke.* The drug does not cure the underlying disorder but helps to facilitate movement and allows *physiotherapy* to be more effective. The drug is taken in either tablet or liquid form.

Side effects of baclofen may include drowsiness and muscle weakness. These effects can be reduced if the dose of the drug is increased gradually under medical supervision until the desired degree of relaxation is achieved.

# Bacteraemia

The presence of *bacteria* in the bloodstream. Bacteraemia commonly occurs for a few hours after minor surgical operations and dental treatment and may also occur in infections such as tonsillitis. The *immune system,* the body's natural defence mechanism, usually prevents the bacteria from multiplying and causing damage. However, in people with abnormal heart valves (due to conditions such as a congenital defect or scarring from rheumatic fever), the bacteria may cause *endocarditis* (inflammation of the heart lining and valves). If bacteraemia affects a person whose immune system is weakened by illness or major surgery, *septicaemia* (an infection of the blood) may develop.

# Bacteria

Single-celled *microorganisms* that are invisible to the naked eye. The singular form of the term is bacterium. Abundant in the air, soil, and water, most bacteria are harmless to humans. Some, such as those that live in the intestine, are beneficial and help to break down food for digestion.

### DISEASE-CAUSING TYPES
Disease-causing bacteria are known as pathogens and are classified, according to shape, into three main groups: *cocci* (spherical); *bacilli* (rod-shaped); and *spirochaetes* or spirilla (spiral-shaped).

Among the wide range of diseases caused by cocci are pneumonia, tonsillitis, bacterial endocarditis (inflammation of the lining inside the heart), meningitis (inflammation of the

---

## CULTURING AND TESTING BACTERIA

Tests to identify bacteria, which are invisible to the naked eye, play an important role in diagnosing diseases. The bacteria to be tested are cultured in the laboratory, on sterile culture plates containing a nutrient gel on which they feed.

**1** *The bacteria are introduced on to a nutrient plate (i.e. agar or blood agar) and placed in an incubator at body temperature.*

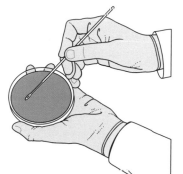

**2** *Any bacteria present multiply rapidly to form visible colonies that can be studied under the microscope and identified by different patterns of growth.*

**3** *To test sensitivity to specific antibiotics, discs of different antibiotics are placed within the colonies of bacteria.*

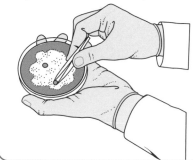

**4** *Any clear areas around each disc indicate that the bacteria are being killed by a particular antibiotic.*

---

membranes surrounding the brain and spinal cord), toxic shock syndrome, and various disorders of the skin.

Diseases that are caused by bacilli include tuberculosis, pertussis (whooping cough), typhoid fever, diphtheria, tetanus, salmonellosis, shigellosis (bacillary dysentery), legionnaires' disease, and botulism.

Bacteria from the third, and smallest, group, the spirochaetes, are responsible for causing syphilis, yaws, leptospirosis, and Lyme disease.

### GROWTH AND MOVEMENT
The bacteria that colonize the human body thrive in warm, moist conditions.

Some of these bacteria are aerobic (they need oxygen to grow and multiply) and are therefore most commonly found on the skin or within the respiratory system. Others are anaerobic, thriving where there is no oxygen, deep within tissue or wounds.

Some types of bacteria are naturally static; if they move around the body at all, they do so only when carried in currents of air or fluid. However, there are also highly motile types of bacteria, such as salmonella, which move through fluids by lashing with their whiplike tails (known as flagella) and can anchor themselves to other cells with filamentous threads called pili.

# BACTERIA

Bacteria are microscopic single-celled organisms that are found in every environment. Some bacteria live in or on our bodies without causing disease. There are thousands of different types of bacterium, but relatively few of these cause disease in humans. Bacteria have a variety of shapes that are broadly classified as cocci (spheres), bacilli (rods), and spirochaetes and spirilla (curved forms).

Sex pilus    Bacterium

## Conjugation

*Bacteria may exchange genes in a process called conjugation. Plasmids, which may contain genes that give the bacteria resistance to antibiotics, are passed through tubes called sex pili.*

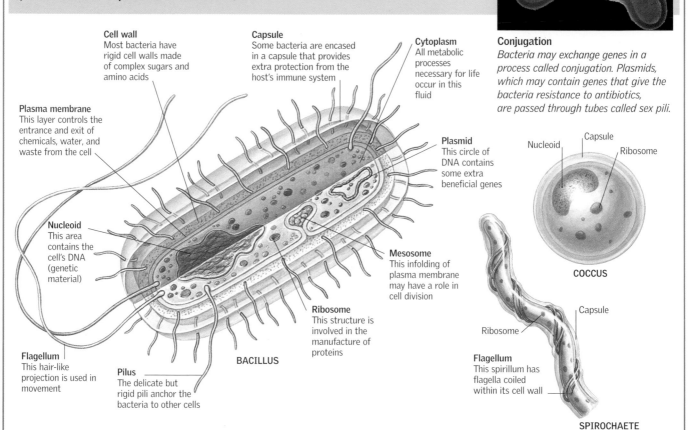

**Cell wall**
Most bacteria have rigid cell walls made of complex sugars and amino acids

**Capsule**
Some bacteria are encased in a capsule that provides extra protection from the host's immune system

**Cytoplasm**
All metabolic processes necessary for life occur in this fluid

**Plasma membrane**
This layer controls the entrance and exit of chemicals, water, and waste from the cell

**Plasmid**
This circle of DNA contains some extra beneficial genes

**Nucleoid**
This area contains the cell's DNA (genetic material)

**Mesosome**
This infolding of plasma membrane may have a role in cell division

**Ribosome**
This structure is involved in the manufacture of proteins

**Flagellum**
This hair-like projection is used in movement

**Pilus**
The delicate but rigid pili anchor the bacteria to other cells

BACILLUS

Nucleoid    Capsule    Ribosome

COCCUS

Capsule

Ribosome

**Flagellum**
This spirillum has flagella coiled within its cell wall

SPIROCHAETE

## Effects of toxins

Some bacteria cause disease by producing poisonous chemicals known as toxins. These chemicals may destroy specific body cells or enter cells and alter their chemical processes. Some toxins are released from bacteria when they die and may cause shock and fever.

**1** *The toxin is released into the body by the bacterium. The toxin attaches to a body cell and is absorbed into the fluid cytoplasm.*

Toxin produced by the bacterium    Body cell

Bacterium

Cytoplasm    Nucleus

**2** *The toxin disrupts normal chemical reactions inside the cell, so that the cell is unable to function and dies.*

Toxin

Dying body cell

## Bacterial invasion of a cell

A few bacteria damage tissues in the human body not by secreting toxins but by directly invading the cells. Once inside body cells, the bacteria reproduce and eventually burst out, rupturing the cell membrane.

**1** *Different bacteria are specifically attracted to certain body cells. Bacteria enter the cell through the membrane and use the cell nutrients.*

Bacterium inside cell    Nucleus

Bacterium

Body cell

**2** *The bacteria multiply rapidly in the cell. They kill the cell by breaking its membrane then spread to other areas of the body.*

Dying body cell

New bacterium breaking out of cell

## REPRODUCTION

Bacteria reproduce by simple cell division, which can occur every few minutes in ideal conditions (exactly the right temperature and sufficient nourishment for all cells).

Some bacteria multiply by each producing a spore (a single new bacterium). Spores, which are protected by a tough membrane, can survive high temperatures, dry conditions, and lack of nourishment.

## HOW BACTERIA ENTER THE BODY

Bacteria can enter the body through the lungs if they are inhaled in infected droplets spread by coughs and sneezes. The digestive tract may become infected if contaminated food is eaten. Some bacteria cause diseases, such as sexually transmitted infections, by entering the genito-urinary system.

Bacteria can also penetrate the skin in various ways: through hair follicles; by way of superficial cuts and abrasions; through burns; and via deep, penetrating wounds.

## HOW BACTERIA CAUSE DISEASE

Some bacteria release poisons (toxins) that are harmful to human cells. The toxins either destroy the cell or disrupt its chemical processes. Less commonly, certain types of bacteria directly enter, and multiply within, body cells, causing tissue damage as they spread.

## THE BODY'S DEFENCES

The body's first defences against disease-causing bacteria are the skin and the *mucous membranes* lining the respiratory tract, the digestive tract, and the genitourinary system.

The eyes are protected by an *enzyme* in tears and the stomach secretes hydrochloric acid, which kills many of the bacteria found in food and water.

If bacteria pass through these barriers, the body's *immune system* responds by sending various types of white blood cell to seek and destroy the bacteria.

Immunity can also be generated by *immunization*. This involves injecting a weakened form of the bacterium or its poison into the body to stimulate an immune response. Immunization is now routine for a number of conditions, including *diphtheria, tetanus,* and some forms of *meningitis*.

## TREATMENT OF BACTERIAL DISEASES

The immune response is sometimes enough to bring about recovery, and mild bacterial infections may not need any treatment. However, *antibiotic drugs* are the main form of treatment for more severe infections. Superficial infected wounds may be treated with *antiseptics*.

Some bacteria, such as *MRSA*, are now becoming resistant to treatment with antibiotics. In these circumstances, bacterial infections can be difficult or even impossible to treat and may be life-threatening. (See also *infectious disease*.)

# Bacterial vaginosis

An infection of the *vagina* that causes a greyish-white discharge and itching. The disorder is due to excessive growth of *bacteria* that normally live in the vagina. Bacterial vaginosis occurs most commonly in sexually active women and is treated with *antibiotic drugs*.

# Bactericidal

A term that is used to describe any substance that kills bacteria. (See also *antibiotic drugs; bacteriostatic*.)

# Bacteriology

The study of *bacteria,* particularly of the types that cause disease. Bacteriology includes techniques used to isolate and identify bacteria from specimens such as a throat swab or urine. Bacteria are identified by their appearance under a microscope, including their response to stains (see *Gram's stain; staining*), and by the use of *culture*. Testing for sensitivity to *antibiotic drugs* may be performed.

# Bacteriostatic

A term used to describe a substance that stops the growth of *bacteria* but does not kill them. (See also *antibiotic drugs; bactericidal*.)

# Bacteriuria

The presence of *bacteria* in the urine. It is common for small, harmless numbers of bacteria to be found in the urine of healthy people. Bacteriuria is of significance only if more than 100,000 bacteria are present in each millilitre of urine, or if 100 white blood cells (pus cells) per millilitre of urine are present (which is an indication of the body's response to the infection).

# Bagassosis

An occupational disease affecting the lungs of workers who handle mouldy bagasse (the fibrous residue of sugar cane after juice extraction). Bagassosis is one cause of allergic *alveolitis,* a reaction of the lungs to inhaled dust containing fungal spores. Symptoms develop four to five hours after inhalation of the dust and may include shortness of breath, wheezing, fever, headache, and cough; typically, they last for about 24 hours. Repeated exposure to dust may lead to permanent lung damage. Protective measures taken by industry have made the disease rare.

# Baker's cyst

A firm, fluid-filled lump behind the knee. A Baker's cyst occurs as a result of increased pressure in the knee joint due to a buildup of fluid. Such a build-up is a feature of disorders such as *rheumatoid arthritis*. The cyst is created by a backward ballooning-out of the synovial membrane covering the knee joint.

**B**

Most Baker's cysts are painless, and some disappear spontaneously, sometimes after many months. Occasionally, a cyst may rupture, causing fluid to seep down between the layers of the calf muscles. This can produce pain and swelling in the calf that may mimic a deep vein thrombosis (see *thrombosis, deep vein*).

Diagnosis of a Baker's cyst is confirmed by *ultrasound scanning*. Treatment is rarely needed, but in a few cases surgery may be performed.

# Balance

The ability to remain upright and move without falling over. Keeping one's balance is a complex process that relies on a constant flow of information to the brain about body position. The integration of all of this information, and continual instructions from the brain, enable the body to make the changes needed to maintain balance.

The brain receives data on body position from various sources: the eyes; the sensory organs (called proprioceptors) in the skin, muscles, and joints; and the three semicircular canals of the labyrinth of the inner *ear*. The part of the brain called the *cerebellum* collates this information and sends instructions to muscles to contract or relax to maintain balance.

### DISORDERS
Balance can be affected by various disorders, particularly inner-ear disorders such as *labyrinthitis* (inflammation of the ear's labyrinth) and *Ménière's disease* (an abnormally high pressure of fluid in the labyrinth). Less commonly, *otitis media* (a disorder of the middle ear) may disturb balance.

Damage to nerve tracts in the spinal cord that carry information from position sensors in the joints and muscles to the brain can also impair balance. This damage to the nerves may result from spinal tumours, circulatory disorders, nerve degeneration due to deficiency of vitamin $B_{12}$, or, rarely, tabes dorsalis (a complication of *syphilis*). A tumour or *stroke* that affects the cerebellum in the brain may cause clumsiness of the arms and legs as well as other features of impaired muscular coordination.

# Balanitis

Inflammation of the foreskin and the glans (head) of the penis. Balanitis results in pain and/or itchiness, and the entire area may be red and moist. Causes of balanitis include bacterial or fungal infection, *phimosis* (tightness of the foreskin), or chemical irritation by contraceptive creams (see contraception) or by laundry products.

Treatment is usually with *antibiotic drugs* or *antifungal drugs* (either applied to the skin as cream or taken orally) and careful washing of the penis and foreskin. If balanitis recurs frequently, or is due to phimosis, *circumcision* (surgical removal of the foreskin) may be recommended.

# Ball-and-socket joint

A highly mobile *joint*, such as the shoulder or hip, in which the ball-shaped end of one bone fits into a cup-shaped cavity in another, allowing movement in all directions.

# Ballismus

Violent jerking and twitching of the limbs that is caused by brain damage within the area below the *thalamus* (a structure that relays sensory information). In most cases, only one side of the body is affected, in which case the condition is known as hemiballismus.

# Balloon angioplasty

See *angioplasty, balloon*.

# Balloon catheter

A flexible tube with a balloon at its tip, which, when inflated, keeps the tube in place or applies pressure to an organ or vessel. One type of balloon catheter is used to drain urine from the bladder (see box, left, and *catheterization, urinary*). Balloon catheters are sometimes used to expand narrowed arteries (see *angioplasty, balloon*). They may also be used to control bleeding from widened veins in the lower part of the oesophagus (known as *oesophageal varices*) before surgery.

# Ballottement

A technique occasionally used during a physical examination (see *examination, physical*) to check the position of an organ, particularly in a fluid-filled area of the body. It involves flicking or tapping the area with the fingers, causing the organ to move up and down. The technique was once widely used to confirm pregnancy; when the wall of the uterus is tapped, the fetus moves away and floats back with a responding tap.

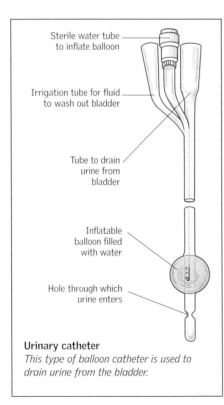

**Urinary catheter**
*This type of balloon catheter is used to drain urine from the bladder.*

**B**

# YOUR BODY: THE SENSE OF BALANCE

The ability to stand upright and move without falling over depends on our sense of balance. Structures in the inner ear, known as the vestibular apparatus, contribute to balance by detecting the position and movements of the head. The vestibular apparatus is composed of three semicircular canals and the two-chambered vestibule.

Semicircular canal

Vestibule

Location

## The role of hair cells

The head's movements are detected by hair cells found in structures called cristae in the semicircular canals and in two structures called maculae in the vestibule.

**Semicircular canal**
The three semicircular canals lie at right angles to each other. When the head turns, fluid in the canals moves, giving information about the speed and direction of motion

**Crista**
Sensory hair cells in the cristae are embedded in gelatinous caps called cupulae

**Vestibular nerve**
Information about position and motion travels along this nerve to the brain

**Macula**
This sensory area contains hair cells that detect the position of the head

**Vestibule**
The two chambers of the fluid-filled vestibule each contain a sensory structure called a macula

B

## Linear movement and static position

The two maculae within the vestibule of the inner ear sense linear movements – for example, when travelling by car or using a lift – and the orientation of the head relative to gravity. Detecting the head's position in relation to gravity helps us, for example, to know instantly which way is up when we dive into deep water.

Sensory hairs | Gelatinous membrane | Hair cell

**Head upright**
*When the head is held upright, the gelatinous membrane of the macula is stable and the hairs on the hair cells remain in an upright position.*

Upright head | Stable macula

Bent hairs | Displaced membrane | Direction of gravity

**Head in tilted position**
*If the head is held in a tilted position, the pull of gravity displaces the gelatinous membrane. The embedded sensory hairs are bent, triggering the hair cells to produce electrical signals.*

Tilted head | Displaced macula

## Rotational movement

Rotational movements of the head are detected by the cristae in the fluid-filled semicircular canals. The three semicircular canals are at right angles to each other, so head rotation in any direction is detected by at least one canal. The information is used both to maintain balance and to keep vision stable when the head moves.

Fluid | Cupula | Sensory hairs | Hair cell

**Head stationary**
*The fluid in the semicircular canals is not moving. The cupula is upright and the hair cells of the crista are not being stimulated.*

Stationary head | Stable cupula

Direction of fluid pressure | Bent hairs

**Head turning**
*As the head turns, the fluid pressure in the semicircular canals displaces the cupula, bending the sensory hairs, which create electrical impulses.*

Turning head | Displaced cupula

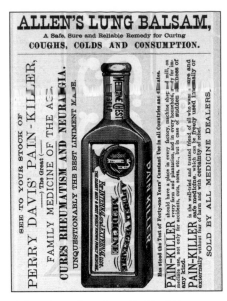

*Balsam is an oily, resinous liquid, which comes from plants such as pine trees. In the past, preparations of balsam were widely used as remedies for coughs, cold, and consumption (tuberculosis).*

## Balsam

An aromatic oily liquid that is obtained from various evergreen trees. Balsam is an *antiseptic* substance and was once also widely used in remedies for respiratory disorders.

## Bandage

A strip or tube of fabric used to keep *dressings* in position, to apply pressure, to control bleeding, or to support a sprain or strain. Roller and tubular bandages are the type most widely used. Tubular gauze bandages require a special applicator and are used mainly for areas that are awkward to bandage, such as a finger. Triangular bandages are used to make *slings*. (See also *wounds*.)

## Banding

A procedure for treating *haemorrhoids* (piles) that are large or are causing particular discomfort. Using a special instrument, a doctor places a rubber band around the base of the haemorrhoid, which causes it to shrink and, eventually, to fall off. Banding is virtually painless and the procedure can be performed in a doctor's surgery.

## Barbiturate drugs

### COMMON DRUGS

•Amobarbital •Butobarbital •Phenobarbital •Secobarbital •Thiopental

A group of sedative drugs that work by depressing activity within the brain. Barbiturate drugs include thiopental, which is very short-acting and is used to induce anaesthesia (see *anaesthesia, general*), and phenobarbital, which is long-acting and is sometimes used as an *anticonvulsant drug* in the treatment of epilepsy. In the past, barbiturates were widely used as *antianxiety drugs* and *sleeping drugs*, but they have been largely replaced by *benzodiazepine drugs* and other nonbarbiturates. Because barbiturates are habit-forming and are widely abused for their sedative effect, they are now classed as *controlled drugs*.

### HOW THEY WORK

The sedative action of barbiturate drugs is produced by the drug molecules blocking the conduction of stimulatory chemical signals between the nerve cells of the brain and reducing the ability of the cells to respond. Barbiturates, especially phenobarbital, also reduce the sensitivity of brain cells to abnormal electrical activity.

### POSSIBLE SIDE EFFECTS

The possible adverse effects of barbiturate drugs include excessive drowsiness, staggering gait, and, in some cases, excitability. An overdose of barbiturates can be fatal, particularly when taken in combination with alcohol, which dangerously increases their depressant effect on the brain (including suppression of the respiratory centre).

Barbiturates are likely to produce *drug dependence* if used for longer than a few weeks, and withdrawal effects, such as sleeplessness and twitching, may then occur when treatment is stopped.

## Barium sulphate

A salt that is used in solution as a *contrast medium* in X-ray examinations of the intestinal tract (see *barium X-ray examinations*).

Barium is opaque to X-rays and is used to view the outline of hollow internal organs, which would otherwise not be visible.

## Barium X-ray examinations

Procedures used to detect and follow the progress of some disorders of the gastrointestinal tract.

Because barium (a metallic element) is opaque to X-rays, it is used to outline organs, such as the stomach,

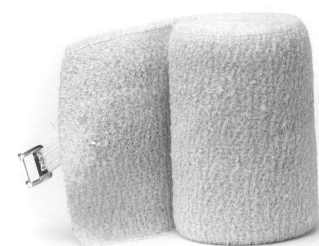

**Bandages are available** *in various sizes and weights. They may be adhesive or made from stretchy fabric so they can be easily wound around joints.*

# BARIUM X-RAY PROCEDURES

Barium X-ray examinations are used to reveal abnormalities or disorders in the upper and lower gastrointestinal tract. Barium swallows are used to investigate the oesophagus, and barium meals are used for the examination of the stomach and duodenum. The large intestine is examined by means of a barium enema.

## BARIUM SWALLOW/MEAL

Barium swallows and meals are used to investigate the upper gastrointestinal tract. No food or drink is permitted for six to nine hours beforehand. At the examination, the patient swallows a glass of barium mixed with a flavoured liquid, or is given a piece of bread or a biscuit soaked in barium if a disorder of the swallowing mechanism is being investigated.

**Taking the X-ray**
*The radiographer takes X-ray pictures while the patient swallows. For a barium swallow, the patient stands; for a barium meal, the patient lies on the table in different positions; for a barium follow-through, the patient lies on the right side and X-rays are taken at intervals until the barium has progressed through the small intestine.*

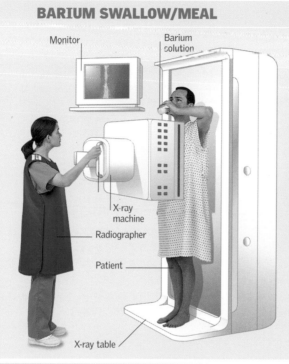

Monitor · Barium solution · Stomach · X-ray machine · Radiographer · Patient · X-ray table · Spine · Tumour

**Barium meal result**
*In this X-ray, the upper part of the stomach at top right (pink) is healthy but there is a tumour in the lower part of the stomach.*

## BARIUM ENEMA

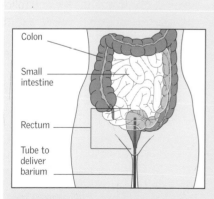

Colon · Small intestine · Rectum · Tube to deliver barium

A barium enema is carried out for examination of the large intestine and rectum. For an examination to be successful, the large intestine needs to be empty and clean because faeces can obscure or simulate a polyp or tumour. For this reason, the patient's intake of food and fluids may be restricted for a few days before the examination, and laxatives are given to make sure that the bowel is empty prior to the procedure.

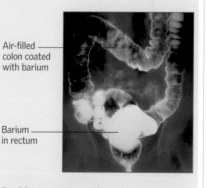

Air-filled colon coated with barium · Barium in rectum

**The procedure**
*The radiographer or radiologist introduces the barium into the patient's intestine via a tube inserted into the rectum. The patient lies on his or her left side while the barium is infused. He or she then turns on to the other side, front, and back, and X-rays are taken.*

**Single-contrast barium enema**
For this procedure, the section of intestine to be examined is filled with liquid barium. Because barium is opaque to X-rays, it provides an outline image that shows up prominent abnormalities such as narrowing.

**Double-contrast result**
*In double-contrast, barium and air are introduced into the tract. The barium forms a film on the tract's inner surface only, providing an image of small surface abnormalities that would not be visible using single-contrast.*

**B**

which are not normally visible on an X-ray image. Barium sulphate mixed with water is passed into the part of the tract requiring examination before X-rays are taken. In some cases, barium X-ray examinations can be used as an alternative to *endoscopy* (internal examination using a rigid or flexible viewing tube).

Barium X-rays may be single- or double-contrast. Single-contrast X-rays use barium sulphate alone. The barium fills the section of the tract under examination and provides an outline image that shows up any prominent abnormalities. In double-contrast barium X-rays, the barium forms a thin film over the inner surface of the tract and the tract is subsequently filled with air so that any small surface abnormalities can be seen

### TYPES OF EXAMINATION

Various types of barium X-ray examination are used to investigate different parts of the gastrointestinal tract. A barium swallow involves drinking a solution of barium; this procedure is used to investigate the swallowing mechanism or the oesophagus. A barium meal is carried out to look at the lower oesophagus, stomach, and duodenum.

A barium follow-through examination can be used to investigate disorders of the small intestine; after barium has been swallowed, a series of X-rays are taken at intervals as the barium travels down the oesophagus to the intestine.

A barium enema can be used to investigate disorders of the large intestine and the rectum; the barium is introduced into the body through a tube inserted in the rectum. Any barium that remains in the intestine may be a cause of constipation. For this reason, it is important to ensure that a patient has a high-fibre diet and drinks plenty of water following a barium examination, until all the barium has passed through. (See also *Barium X-ray procedures* box, on previous page.)

# Barotrauma

Damage or pain, mainly affecting the middle *ear* and the facial *sinuses*, that is caused by changes in surrounding air pressure. Air travellers are at the greatest risk of barotrauma, but scuba divers face similar problems.

### CAUSE

Aircraft cabin pressure decreases as the plane ascends and increases as it descends. As the aircraft ascends, the ears may seem to "pop" as the air in the middle ear expands and is expelled via the eustachian tubes, which connect the middle ear to the back of the throat. On descent, the higher pressure may push the eardrum inwards and cause pain.

### SYMPTOMS

Minor pressure damage in the middle ear may cause pain, hearing loss, and *tinnitus* (ringing in the ears) for a few days; damage in the facial sinuses may also cause pain, and possibly a discharge of mucus or blood.

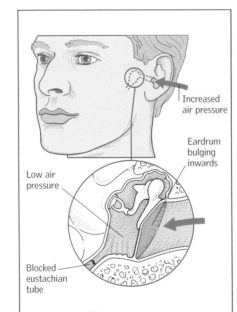

**Mechanism of barotrauma**
*The diagram above shows the location of the middle ear and the pressure changes that occur when the eustachian tube is blocked and there is an increase in surrounding air pressure.*

Symptoms usually wear off within hours or days, but treatment may be needed if they worsen or persist. Large changes in pressure can rupture the eardrum (see *eardrum, perforated*).

### PREVENTION

Barotrauma can be avoided by vigorous swallowing or by forcibly breathing out with the mouth closed and the nose pinched, which is known as the Valsalva manoeuvre. This action serves to equalize the internal and external pressures in the middle ear and sinuses.

If the eustachian tubes are blocked, as commonly occurs with a cold, use of a nasal spray containing a *decongestant drug* is recommended shortly before the descent of the aircraft. Anyone with a severe head cold should avoid air travel if possible. Infants should be breast- or bottle-fed during descent to encourage swallowing. (See also *aviation medicine*; *scuba-diving medicine*.)

# Barrel chest

A prominent, rounded chest that is sometimes the result of lung distension in people with longstanding *emphysema* (enlarged air sacs in the lungs). Lung distension leads to an increase in distance between the front and back of the chest, thereby resulting in a change in the shape of the chest wall.

# Barrett's oesophagus

A complication of long-term gastro-oesophageal reflux (see *acid reflux*), in which the cells that line the lower part of the oesophagus are replaced by cells that are normally found in the stomach. People with Barrett's oesophagus are at increased risk of developing cancer of the oesophagus (see *oesophagus, cancer of*). The condition may be monitored regularly by *endoscopy* (internal examination

# SELF-HELP: BAROTRAUMA

The feeling of "popping ears" is common during air travel, scuba-diving, or even when you travel up or down steep hills in a car. It is due to a difference in pressure between the outside environment and your middle ear, which makes your eardrum bulge and may cause pain, a muffled feeling, ringing in your ears, and temporary hearing loss. Normally, pressures are kept equal by air flowing in and out of the middle ear via the eustachian tubes, which link the middle ear to the nose and throat, but during rapid ascent or descent the tubes are too narrow to cope. Babies and young children have short, narrow tubes and are particularly prone to popping ears. Your ears are also more likely to pop if you have a blocked nose.

There are several steps that you can take to help equalize the pressure in your ears. The discomfort of popping ears usually disappears 3–5 hours after air pressure has stabilized.

- On a plane, chew gum or suck boiled sweets when you are ascending or descending rapidly.

- Swallowing frequently with your mouth open or yawning helps to equalize the pressure.

- You can use a simple technique to unblock your ears (see practical technique, below).

- If you are travelling with a baby, try breastfeeding or bottle-feeding while the plane is ascending or descending, or let your baby suck a dummy. Give your baby plenty of fluids to drink during travel.

- If you are particularly susceptible to popping ears, take a decongestant before you travel (see drug remedies, below).

- If you have a cold, an ear infection, or sinusitis, try to avoid air travel. If you must fly, use a decongestant. If you have hay fever when you fly, take an antihistamine (see drug remedies, below). Don't scuba-dive if you have any of these conditions.

## DRUG REMEDIES

Decongestants, available as drops, sprays, and tablets, shrink the membranes lining the nasal passages. When you fly, use a decongestant an hour before you take off, and repeat as necessary, following the instructions supplied with the product.

Antihistamines will relieve a blocked or runny nose caused by hay fever for the duration of your flight. Take a non-sedative antihistamine before travelling. Repeat as necessary, according to the instructions on the pack.

## SEEK MEDICAL ADVICE

Arrange to see your doctor if:
- Your ears are very painful.
- Symptoms don't subside within 3–5 hours of returning to normal air pressure
- You have a discharge from your ear.
- You have persistent hearing loss

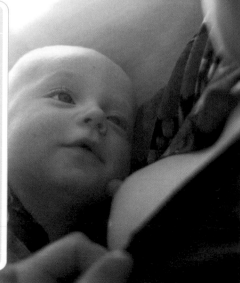

**Feeding your baby** *when landing or taking off can help to prevent your baby from discomfort due to popping ears. Always ensure your baby has plenty to drink during the flight.*

## PRACTICAL TECHNIQUE

Try the following action to relieve discomfort and unblock your ears. You may need to do this several times during ascent or descent.

- Begin by firmly pinching both of your nostrils closed with your index finger and thumb.

- Breathe in through your mouth. Then close your mouth, hold your nose tightly, and gently blow into your nostrils until your ears pop.

**Blowing into your nostrils**
*Be careful not to blow too hard as you could damage your eardrums.*

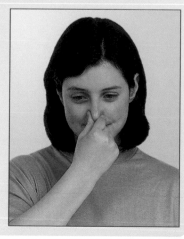

using a viewing instrument) of the oesophagus.

# Barrier cream

A cream that is used to protect the skin against the effects of irritant substances and excessive exposure to water. (See also *sunscreens*.)

# Barrier method

A method of preventing pregnancy by blocking the passage of sperm to the uterus (see *contraception, barrier methods of*). An example of a barrier method is the use of a condom or a diaphragm.

# Barrier nursing

The nursing technique by which a patient with an infectious disease is prevented from infecting other people (see *isolation*). In reverse barrier nursing, a patient with reduced ability to fight infections (for example, because of an *immunodeficiency disorder* or following certain types of surgery) is protected against outside infection. (See also *aseptic technique*.)

# Bartholinitis

An infection of the Bartholin's glands at the entrance to the *vagina*. The disorder, which may be due to a

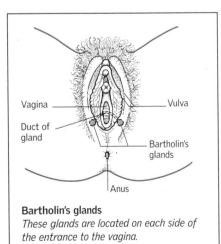

**Bartholin's glands**
*These glands are located on each side of the entrance to the vagina.*

*sexually transmitted infection* such as *gonorrhoea*, causes an intensely painful red swelling at the opening of the gland ducts. Treatment is with *antibiotic drugs*, *analgesic drugs*, and warm baths.

Bartholinitis sometimes leads to the formation of an abscess (Bartholin's abscess) or a painless cyst, known as a Bartholin's cyst, which may become infected. Abscesses are drained under general anaesthesia (see *anaesthesia, general*). Recurrent abscesses or infected cysts may require surgery to convert the duct into an open pouch (see *marsupialization*) or remove the gland completely.

# Basal cell carcinoma

A type of skin cancer, also known as a rodent ulcer or BCC, that occurs most commonly on the face or neck, but can affect any part of the body. The cells of the tumour closely resemble, and are possibly derived from, cells in the basal (innermost) skin layer.

Basal cell carcinoma is caused by skin damage from the ultraviolet radiation in sunlight. Fair-skinned people over the age of 50 are most commonly affected by this form of cancer; dark-skinned people are protected by the larger amount of *melanin* (a pigment that absorbs ultraviolet radiation) in their skin. The incidence of basal cell carcinoma is much higher among people living in sunny climates, especially those who have outdoor occupations; in parts of the US and Australia, over half the white population has had a basal cell carcinoma by the age of 75.

### SYMPTOMS
The majority of basal cell carcinomas occur on the face, often at the side of an eye or on the nose. It starts as a small, flat nodule and grows slowly, eventually breaking down at the centre to form a shallow ulcer with raised edges.

Diagnosis is confirmed through a biopsy (removal of a small sample of cells for microscopic analysis). Without treatment, the tumour gradually

## BASAL CELL CARCINOMA

The most common type of skin cancer, basal cell carcinoma is also the least dangerous because it usually remains localized and rarely spreads to other parts of the body. This cancer should not be left untreated because it can destroy bone and surrounding skin.

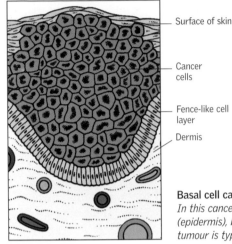
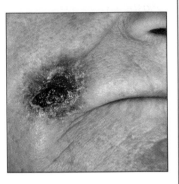

Surface of skin
Cancer cells
Fence-like cell layer
Dermis

**Basal cell carcinoma**
*In this cancer, abnormal cells grow in the outer skin (epidermis), bordered by a fence-like layer of cells. The tumour is typically firm and pearly-looking.*

invades and destroys the surrounding tissues, but it virtually never spreads to other parts of the body.

### TREATMENT
Treatment of basal cell carcinoma is usually with surgery (or in some cases *radiotherapy*) and is often completely successful.

*Plastic surgery* may also be required, however, depending on the size and site of the tumour.

### PREVENTION
The risk of developing this form of skin cancer can be reduced by avoiding overexposure to strong sunlight, by using *sunscreens*, and by wearing protective clothing such as sun hats.

People who have previously had a basal cell carcinoma may develop further tumours and should be especially alert to any new changes in their skin. (See also *melanoma, malignant*; *squamous cell carcinoma*; *sunlight, adverse effects of*.)

## Basal ganglia

Paired nerve cell clusters deep within the cerebrum (the main mass of the *brain*) and the upper part of the brainstem.

The basal ganglia play a vital part in producing smooth, continuous muscular actions and in stopping and starting movement.

Any disease or degeneration affecting the basal ganglia and their connections may lead to the appearance of involuntary movements, trembling, and weakness, as occur in *Parkinson's disease*.

## Basal metabolic rate (BMR)

The rate at which energy is used by the body just to maintain vital functions. Vital functions include breathing, circulation, and digestion. (See also *energy requirements*; *metabolism*).

## Base pair

Part of a *DNA* molecule comprising two chemicals known as nucleotide bases that are linked together by means of hydrogen bonds. A base pair forms one "rung" of the DNA "ladder". There are only two possible pairings of the four bases: guanine always pairs with cytosine and adenine with thymine. The sequence of base pairs in each DNA chain provides the code for the activities of the cell (see *genetic code*). (See also *nucleic acids*.)

## Basic life support

Resuscitation techniques that may be performed by a first aider (see *rescue breathing*; *cardiopulmonary resuscitation*). If basic life support measures fail to restore a normal heartbeat and spontaneous breathing, *advanced life support* must then be administered by medical personnel.

## Basilar membrane

A membrane within the cochlea (the inner *ear* structure containing the receptor for hearing). Sound waves cause the basilar membrane to vibrate, stimulating sensory hair cells to send electrical signals to the brain.

## Basophil

A type of *white blood cell* that plays a part in inflammatory and allergic reactions.

**The BCG vaccination** *gives immunity against tuberculosis. The vaccine is administered at 10 to 14 years old and sometimes shortly after birth.*

## Bates method

See box, page 178.

## Batten's disease

One of a group of hereditary metabolic diseases (see *metabolism, inborn errors of*) to which *Tay–Sachs disease* also belongs. In Batten's disease, abnormal fatty substances accumulate in the cells of the *nervous system*, causing progressive dementia, worsening seizures, and loss of vision. Symptoms of the condition usually first appear during early childhood.

There is no known treatment for Batten's disease, which is generally fatal during childhood.

## Bazin's disease

A rare disorder, mainly affecting young women, in which tender swellings develop under the skin in the calves. In most cases no cause can be found, although Bazin's disease may sometimes be linked to *tuberculosis*.

**B**

## THE BATES METHOD

Devised at the beginning of the 20th century by Dr. William H. Bates, a US ophthalmologist, the Bates method aims to enhance eyesight without the aid of lenses or surgery. Dr. Bates argued that perfect vision was the product of perfectly relaxed eyes, unconsciously controlled, and that misuse of the eyes accounted for many vision defects. He believed that eyes could be re-educated using a series of simple exercises. Practitioners of the Bates method claim that these exercises are of benefit to people of all ages, however good or poor their eyesight.

The Bates method of "vision education" was developed early in the 20th century by New York ophthalmologist Dr. William H. Bates. He believed that bad habits and tension affecting the eye muscles and optic nerves accounted for many vision defects, which could be corrected using eye exercises. Although initially dismissed by doctors, Dr. Bates' theories attracted followers allover the world, among them Margaret Darst Corbett, the US Bates teacher whose pupil, British writer Aldous Huxley, claimed amazing results.

### Consulting a practitioner

The practitioner assesses your eyesight and may suggest 6–10 weekly sessions. You are taught simple eye exercises, to be practised daily. Dr. Bates claimed that bad habits, such as staring, "switch off" the eyes' ability constantly to adjust and focus on an image (a process of "central fixation"). Exercises, he believed, could re-educate the eye and help achieve "optimum" central fixation. He taught patients to relax the optic nerve and eye muscles, and use the powers of memory and imagination to improve co-ordination between the eyes and the brain. Advice on breathing, relaxation, diet and exercise may also be given, since Dr. Bates claimed that lifestyle factors could affect vision capability. Artificial light and vdu screens, which encourage staring, are thought to make eyesight worse.

### Evidence and research

Most trials were carried out in the early 20th century by Dr. Bates. Anecdotal evidence suggests that the method can help improve eyesight, but there have been no recent clinical trials to confirm this.

### Medical opinion

Doctors recognize that vision involves the use of eye muscles and instinctive visual skills, and acknowledge that eye exercises may sometimes improve sight. However, since the Bates method requires a certain amount of perseverance, and improvement may not be dramatic, it is not seen as a substitute for lenses or surgery.

Focus 10–12 times on one pencil, then on the other

The pencil on which you are not focusing will appear double

**Focusing**: to improve focusing, hold one pencil at arm's length and one 15 cm (6 in) in front of you. Focus on one, blink, then focus on the other.

### PRECAUTIONS

- Consult your doctor and a trained teacher if you have glaucoma or cataracts.
- Do not perform eye exercises while wearing glasses or contact lenses.

## B-cell

See *B-lymphocyte*.

## BCG vaccination

A vaccine that gives immunity against *tuberculosis*. The BCG vaccine is prepared from an artificially weakened strain of bovine (cattle) tubercle bacilli, the rod-shaped *bacteria* that are responsible for causing tuberculosis. The letters BCG stand for "bacille Calmette–Guérin", after the two men who developed the tuberculosis vaccine.

### WHY IT IS DONE

The BCG vaccine is given to people who are at risk of tuberculosis and to those whose tuberculin test is negative, indicating that they are likely to have no immunity to the disease. People at risk include health workers, contacts of people with tuberculosis, and immigrants from countries where there is a high rate of tuberculosis. Infants born to immigrants in this category are immunized, without having a tuberculin test, within a few days of birth. The vaccine is also recommended for children aged 10 to 14 years for whom the tuberculin test is negative.

### HOW IT IS DONE

The vaccine is usually injected into the upper arm. About six weeks later, a small pustule appears. This normally heals completely, leaving a small scar, but can occasionally develop into a chronic *ulcer* (open sore).

## Becker's muscular dystrophy

A type of *muscular dystrophy*.

## Beclometasone

A *corticosteroid drug* that is used in the treatment of *asthma* and hay fever (see *rhinitis, allergic*). When prescribed as a nasal spray, beclometasone controls the symptoms of these conditions by reducing inflammation and the production of mucus in the lining of the nose. Prescribed as an inhaler for the treatment of asthma, the drug reduces inflammation of the airways, thereby controlling wheezing and coughing.

Beclometasone is often given with *bronchodilator drugs* in the management of asthma. A severe asthma attack may require the dose to be increased. The action of beclometasone is slow, however, and its full effect takes several days to occur. Possible adverse effects of the drug include hoarseness, throat irritation, and, on rare occasions, fungal infections in the mouth.

Beclometasone is also prescribed in the form of a cream or as an ointment to treat inflammation of the skin resulting from *eczema*.

# Becquerel

A unit of radioactivity.

# Bed bath

A method of washing a bedridden person. A small area is washed and dried at a time, while the rest of the body is kept covered to prevent chilling.

# Bedbug

A flat, wingless, brown insect that is about 5 mm long and 3 mm wide. Bedbugs live in furniture and furnishings, especially in beds and carpets, emerging at night to feed on humans by sucking their blood. Bedbugs are not known to transmit disease, but their bites are itchy and they may develop into sores that become infected.

# Bedpan

A metal, plastic, or fibre container into which a patient can defaecate or urinate without getting out of bed.

# Bed rest

A term used to describe periods spent in bed. Bed rest is sometimes part of the treatment for certain illnesses, such as rheumatic fever, and for some types of injury, such as a fractured vertebra.

Prolonged bed rest carries risks such as muscle wasting, bedsores, and development of blood clots in the legs. Bed rest was once considered an essential part of the treatment of many common conditions, but it is now avoided when possible. Patients are usually encouraged to be mobile as soon as they are able following illness or surgery.

# Bedridden

A term used to describe a person who is unable to leave bed due to illness or injury.

People most likely to be bedridden are the very elderly, the terminally ill, and those paralysed as the result of an accident.

# Bedsore

Also known as a decubitus ulcer or pressure sore, an ulcer that forms on the skin of patients who are unconscious or immobile. Common sites for bedsores include the shoulders, elbows, lower back, hips, buttocks, ankles, and heels.

### CAUSES
Bedsores may develop following a *stroke* or *spinal injuries* that result in loss of sensation. Incontinence (see *incontinence, urinary*), if it results in constantly wet skin, may also be a causative factor.

### SYMPTOMS
Bedsores start as red, painful areas that become purple before the skin starts to break down, producing open sores. At this stage, the sores may become infected and take a long time to heal.

### TREATMENT AND PREVENTION
Deep, chronic *ulcers* may require treatment with *antibiotic drugs* and, in

**B**

---

## SELF-HELP: PREVENTING BEDSORES

Once a bedsore has developed it will heal only if pressure on it is minimized, so good nursing care of a bedridden or immobile patient is crucial. The patient's position should be changed at least every two hours; and it is important to wash and dry pressure areas carefully, especially if there is incontinence. Barrier creams can be used for additional protection.

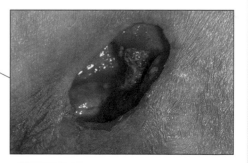

**Common sites**
*These include the shoulders, elbows, lower back, hips and buttocks, knees, ankles, and heels.*

## BEHAVIOURAL PROBLEMS IN CHILDREN

If a child has persistent problems with basic aspects of daily living, such as sleeping, eating, and toilet training, the effects can be very disruptive to the family. Behaviour problems that commonly occur in children can often be overcome with simple self-help measures, and most will eventually cease as a child matures. Only rarely do such behaviours indicate underlying psychological problems.

If a child's behaviour is causing problems *a parent or carer should try to offer support and reassurance, and encourage the child to talk about any difficulties she may be having at play or at school.*

- **Babies up to 18 months**
  Sleeping and feeding difficulties, colic, crying

- **Toddlers and children 1–4 years**
  Head-banging, tantrums, biting, breath-holding attacks, separation anxiety, poor social interaction, difficulty in changing from one activity to another, toilet training problems

- **Early childhood 4–8 years**
  Nail-biting, thumb-sucking, aggression, clinginess, anxiety about illness and death, nightmare, enuresis

- **Middle childhood/adolescence 9–18 years**
  Lying, stealing, smoking, truancy, disobedience, aggression, low achievement in school, drug or alcohol use, running away, sexual promiscuity

some cases, *plastic surgery*. Good nursing care, including changing the patient's position regularly, skin care, protection of vulnerable areas, and use of cushions and special mattresses, should prevent bedsores from developing in most cases.

## Bedwetting

The common name for poor bladder control at night (see *enuresis, nocturnal*).

## Behavioural problems in children

Behavioural problems range from mild and short-lived periods of unacceptable behaviour, which are common in most children, to more severe problems such as conduct disorders and refusal to go to school. Behavioural problems may occasionally occur in any child; specialist management is called for when the problems become frequent and disrupt school and/or family life. Some behavioural problems can occur whatever the family or home situation of the child. In some cases, however, stressful external events, such as moving home or parental divorce, may produce periods of problem behaviour.

Behavioural problems that are common in young children include sleeping problems, such as waking repeatedly in the night. In toddlers, *breath-holding attacks*, *tantrums*, separation anxiety, and *head-banging* are problems best dealt with by a

consistent and controlled approach. Problems with *toilet-training* are usually avoided if the training is delayed until the child is physically and emotionally ready.

In children between the ages of four and eight years, minor behavioural problems, such as *thumb-sucking* and nail-biting, clinginess, bedwetting (see *enuresis, nocturnal*), and disruption during the night due to *nightmares*, are so common as to be almost normal. Such problems are best dealt with by using a positive approach that concentrates on rewarding good behaviour. In most cases, the child grows out of the problem, but medical help from a child guidance counsellor or a child psychiatrist may occasionally be needed.

## Behaviour therapy

A collection of techniques, based on psychological theory, that are used to change abnormal behaviour or to treat anxiety. Behaviour therapy is based on two main ideas: that repeated exposure to a feared experience under safe conditions will render it less threatening, and that desirable behaviour can be encouraged by using a system of rewards, often self-administered.

### TYPES

Specific behaviour therapy techniques include exposure therapy (also known as desensitization), flooding, response prevention, and modelling.

**EXPOSURE THERAPY** A technique that is commonly used to treat phobic disorders, such as *agoraphobia* (a fear of open spaces and/or public places), animal phobias, and fear of flying. It consists of exposing the patient to the cause of the anxiety in stages: for example, the therapist may accompany an agoraphobic patient on a short journey. At the same time, the patient is taught to cope with anxiety symptoms by using relaxation techniques. The intensity of the exposure is increased, until eventually,

**B**

he or she is able to deal with the full situation.

**FLOODING** In flooding, the patient is confronted directly and for a lengthy period with the anxiety-provoking stimulus. He or she is supported by the therapist until the fear is reduced.

This technique can be emotionally traumatic and is now used less commonly.

**RESPONSE PREVENTION** The patient is prevented from carrying out an obsessional task. For example, someone with a handwashing compulsion is prevented from carrying out the washing rituals. This technique is used in combination with other methods.

**MODELLING** In this approach, the therapist acts as a model for the patient, performing the anxiety-provoking activity first, and encouraging the patient to copy.

# Behaviour, types A and B

Behaviours characteristic of two personality types described in the early 1970s, when studies were performed to examine the behaviour patterns of people with coronary artery disease.

It was proposed that a particular behaviour pattern (called Type A) was associated with increased

vulnerability to stress-related illnesses, such as *hypertension* (high blood pressure). Type A personalities are said to feel constantly under pressure to perform many tasks at the same time, and to be competitive and self-critical.

They are also impatient and easily irritated by others. In contrast to this, people with Type B personalities are said to be calmer and more relaxed.

# Belching

The noisy return of air from the stomach through the mouth. Swallowing air is usually an unconscious habit, which may result from eating or drinking too much or too quickly, or both.

Occasionally, belching may help to alleviate discomfort that is caused by indigestion.

# Belladonna

An extract of the deadly nightshade plant that has, since ancient times, been used medicinally.

Belladonna contains *alkaloids* (substances containing nitrogen), such as *atropine*, that are used as *antispasmodic drugs* to treat gastrointestinal disturbances. (See also *anticholinergic drugs*.)

**The deadly nightshade plant** *is the source of belladonna, a highly poisonous chemical from which medically useful substances, such as atropine, can be extracted.*

# Bell's palsy

The most common form of *facial palsy* (facial muscle weakness).

# Bence–Jones protein

An abnormal protein found in the urine of people with *multiple myeloma*, which is a cancer affecting one type of cell in the bone marrow.

# Bendroflumethiazide

A thiazide *diuretic drug* that is used to treat *hypertension* (high blood pressure) and *heart failure*.

# Bends

The nonmedical term for *decompression sickness*. The term is used especially to refer to the severe bone and joint pains that are a common symptom in divers who rise to the surface too rapidly.

# Benign

A term used to describe a disease that is relatively harmless. When used to refer to tumours, benign means noncancerous tumours that do not invade or destroy local tissues and do not spread to other sites within the body.

# Benign prostatic hyperplasia (BPH)

A medical term for noncancerous enlargement of the prostate gland (see *prostate, enlarged*).

# Bennett's fracture

A fracture of the base of the thumb, which is often accompanied by partial dislocation of the joint.

## Benorilate

A *nonsteroidal anti-inflammatory drug* (NSAID) that contains *aspirin* and *paracetamol*. Benorilate is mainly used to relieve joint pain and stiffness in *osteoarthritis* and *rheumatoid arthritis*. Side effects of benorilate are not usually serious, but the aspirin in the drug may cause nausea, indigestion, or bleeding from the stomach lining.

## Benzalkonium chloride

A preservative that is widely used in eye-drops and products such as cosmetics and mouth washes.

## Benzocaine

A local anaesthetic (see *anaesthesia, local*) commonly used as an ingredient in over-the-counter preparations for relieving the pain of conditions such as *mouth ulcers* and *sore throat*.

## Benzodiazepine drugs

### COMMON DRUGS

**SLEEPING DRUGS** •Flunitrazepam •Flurazepam •Loprazolam •Lormetazepam •Nitrazepam •Temazepam
**SEDATIVES** •Alprazolam •Chlordiazepoxide •Clorazepate •Diazepam •Lorazepam •Oxazepam

A group of sedative drugs given for short periods either as *sleeping drugs* for *insomnia* or to control the symptoms of *anxiety* (see *tranquillizer drugs*).

Common benzodiazepine drugs include diazepam, which is used as a tranquillizer, and nitrazepam, which is used to relieve insomnia.

Benzodiazepine drugs are also used in the management of alcohol withdrawal and in the short-term control of an epileptic seizure.

**After the death of a loved one**, *there is a period of bereavement, in which emotions fluctuate between numbness, anger, despair, and possibly depression.*

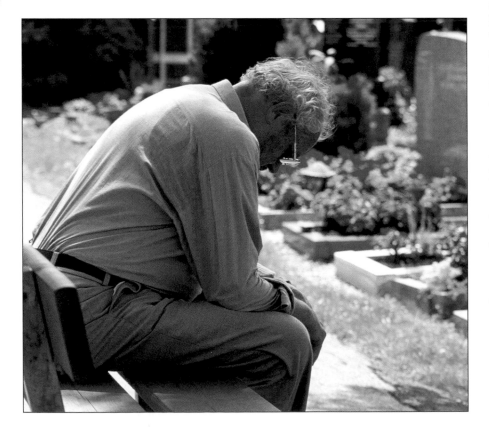

### HOW THEY WORK

Benzodiazepine drugs promote sleep and relieve anxiety by interfering with chemical activity in the brain and nervous system. This reduces the communication between nerve cells and depresses brain activity.

### POSSIBLE ADVERSE EFFECTS

Adverse effects of benzodiazepines include excessive daytime drowsiness, dizziness, and forgetfulness. Unsteadiness and slowed reactions may also occur. If taken with alcohol, benzodiazepines may increase the alcohol's effect to a dangerous extent.

After as little as two weeks, users of a benzodiazepine drug may become psychologically and physically dependent on the drug. For this reason, most doctors are now reluctant to prescribe the drugs unless they are absolutely necessary, and then only for a maximum of three weeks.

When benzodiazepine treatment is stopped suddenly, withdrawal symptoms, such as anxiety, restlessness, and nightmares may occur. People who have been taking benzodiazepine drugs long term need to have them gradually withdrawn over the course of several months to prevent withdrawal symptoms. Benzodiazepines are sometimes abused for their sedative effects.

## Benzoyl peroxide

An *antiseptic agent* used in the treatment of *acne* and fungal skin infections (see *fungal infections*). In acne, benzoyl peroxide also works by removing the surface layer of skin, thereby unblocking sebaceous glands.

## Benzylpenicillin

A type of *penicillin drug* that is given by injection.

## Bereavement

The emotional reaction following the death of a loved one. The expression of grief is individual to each person, but there are recognized stages of bereavement, each of which is characterized by a particular attitude.

## STAGES OF BEREAVEMENT

In the first stage of bereavement, which may last from three days to three months, there is often a feeling of numbness and an unwillingness to recognize the death

These emotions are defence mechanisms against admitting, and therefore accepting, the loss and the associated pain. Often, the reality of the death does not penetrate completely at this time, and many people continue to behave as though the dead person were still alive.

Hallucinations, in which the deceased person is seen or sensed, are a common experience among the recently bereaved. This sensation can be quite comforting for some people, but others may find it disturbing.

Once the numbness wears off, the person may be overwhelmed by feelings of anxiety, anger, and despair that can develop into a depressive illness (see *depression*).

Gastrointestinal disturbances, insomnia, malaise, agitation, and tearfulness are also common.

Gradually, but usually within two years, the bereaved person adjusts to the loss and begins to look more towards the future.

This process can involve periods of pain and despair, alternating with periods of enthusiasm and interest.

## SUPPORT AND COUNSELLING

Family and friends can often provide the support a bereaved person needs. Outside help is sometimes required and may be given by a social worker, health visitor, member of the clergy, or self-help group.

For some people, when depression, apathy, and lethargy impede their chances of recovery, specialized counselling or psychotherapy is necessary. (See also *stillbirth*.)

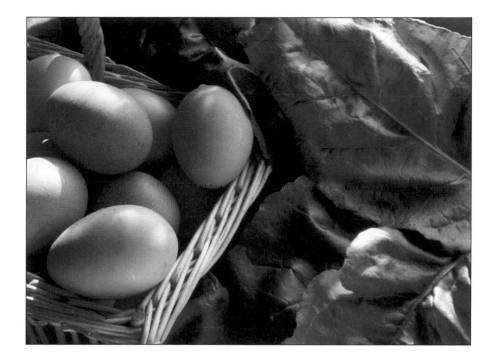

# Beriberi

A nutritional disorder resulting from a lack of thiamine (vitamin B1) in the diet. Thiamine, found in wholemeal cereals, meat, peas, spinach, eggs, fish, and nuts, is essential for the metabolism of carbohydrates. Without it, the brain, the nerves, and the muscles (including the heart muscle) are not able to function properly. In developed countries, the illness is seen only in people who are starving or those who have an extremely restricted diet, such as alcoholics.

## SYMPTOMS AND SIGNS

There are two forms of the illness: "dry" and "wet" beriberi. In dry beriberi, thiamine deficiency mainly affects the nerves and skeletal muscles. The symptoms include numbness, a burning sensation in the legs, and muscle wasting. In severe cases, the affected person becomes virtually paralysed, emaciated, and bedridden.

In wet beriberi, the main problem is heart failure (the inability of the heart to maintain efficient pumping of blood around the body). This in turn causes oedema (swelling caused by fluid accumulation) in the legs and

**Vitamin B$_1$ (thiamine)** *is needed for normal functioning of the body. A deficiency of the vitamin can cause diseases such as beriberi, which affects the nervous system. Good sources of vitamin B$_1$ are peas, spinach, liver, beef, nuts, wholemeal bread, soya beans, eggs, and fish.*

sometimes also in the trunk and face. Other symptoms of wet beriberi include poor appetite, rapid pulse, and breathlessness.

Without treatment, heart failure worsens and can lead to death.

## TREATMENT

Beriberi is treated with thiamine, given either orally or by injection, which usually brings about a complete cure. A permanent improvement in diet is also required to prevent recurrence.

# Bernard–Soulier syndrome

A genetic disorder in which platelets (the blood cells responsible for initiating blood clotting) do not function properly.

The syndrome is characterized by abnormal bleeding in the skin and internal organs.

**B**

# Berry aneurysm

An abnormal swelling that occurs at the junction of *arteries* supplying the brain. Berry aneurysms are usually due to a congenital (present at birth) weakness in the artery wall. They may occasionally rupture, which results in a *subarachnoid haemorrhage.* (See also *aneurysm; intracranial aneurysm.*)

# Berylliosis

An occupational disease caused by the inhalation of dust or fumes containing beryllium, a metallic element that is used in high-technology industries such as nuclear energy, electronics, and aerospace. Short exposure to high concentrations of beryllium may lead to an episode of severe *pneumonitis* (lung inflammation). Exposure to smaller concentrations over a number of years may lead to permanent damage to the lungs and the liver.

Treatment with *corticosteroid drugs* can reduce damage to the lungs. In most cases, the introduction of safe working practices prevents exposure to dangerous levels of beryllium.

# Best's disease

A *genetic disorder* in which the macula (part of the light-sensitive retina at the back of the eye) is abnormal. The disorder is congenital (present from birth) and results in progressive loss of vision.

# Beta-blocker drugs

### COMMON DRUGS

CARDIOSELECTIVE • Atenolol • Betaxolol • Bisoprolol • Celiprolol • Metoprolol
NONCARDIOSELECTIVE • Acebutolol • Carvedilol • Labetolol • Nadolol • Oxprenolol • Pindolol • Propranolol • Sotalol • Timolol

A group of drugs, also known as beta-adrenergic blocking agents, prescribed principally to treat heart and circulatory disorders such as angina pectoris (pain in the chest due to an

## HOW BETA-BLOCKERS WORK

Beta-blockers block specific sites on body tissues where neurotransmitters (chemicals released from nerve endings) bind. These sites are called beta receptors, and there are two types. beta$_1$ receptors, found in heart tissue, and beta$_2$ receptors, found in the lungs, blood vessels, and other tissues. At these receptors, two chemicals, adrenaline (epinephrine) and noradrenaline (norepinephrine), are released from nerve endings in the sympathetic nervous system, the part of the involuntary nervous system that enables the body to deal with stress, anxiety, and exercise. These neurotransmitters bind to beta receptors to increase the force and speed of the heartbeat, to dilate the airways to increase air flow to the lungs, and to dilate blood vessels.

Cardioselective beta-blockers bind predominantly to beta$_1$ receptors; noncardioselective beta-blockers bind to both types. Beta-blockers slow the heart rate and reduce the force of contraction of heart muscle. These effects can be used to slow a fast heart rate and regulate abnormal rhythms.

Beta-blockers prevent attacks of angina pectoris by reducing the work of the heart muscle and therefore the heart's oxygen requirement. High blood pressure is reduced because the rate and force at which the heart pumps blood into the circulation is lowered.

The effect of blocking beta receptors on muscles elsewhere in the body is to reduce the muscle tremor of anxiety and an overactive thyroid gland. Beta-blockers may help to reduce the frequency of migraine attacks by preventing the dilation of blood vessels surrounding the brain, which is what causes the headache. In glaucoma they lower pressure in the eye by reducing fluid production in the eyeball.

#### Normal
*Adrenaline (epinephrine) and noradrenaline (norepinephrine) can be released either from the adrenal gland or from sympathetic nerve endings. They bind to beta$_1$ and beta$_2$ receptors in tissues around the body.*

#### Cardioselective beta-blockers
*Cardioselective beta-blockers occupy predominantly B$_1$ receptors, preventing adrenaline and noradrenaline from binding to them. This reduces the stimulating action of adrenaline and noradrenaline on heart tissue. Cardioselective beta-blockers do not block B$_2$ receptors, thereby allowing adrenaline (epinephrine)/noradrenaline (norepinephrine) to act on other tissues around the body.*

#### Noncardioselective beta-blockers
*Noncardioselective beta-blockers occupy both B$_1$ and B$_2$ receptors, reducing the stimulating action of adrenaline (epinephrine) and noradrenaline (norepinephrine) on tissues around the body.*

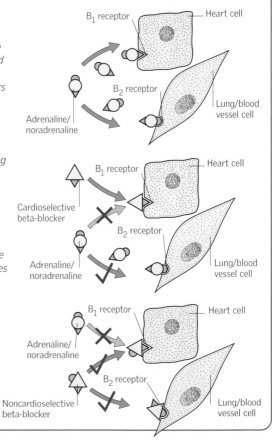

insufficient supply of blood to the heart muscle) and *hypertension* (high blood pressure). The drugs block the effects of the *sympathetic nervous system*, which releases *adrenaline* (epinephrine) and *noradrenaline* (norepinephrine) at nerve endings known as beta receptors.

There are two types of beta receptor: $beta_1$ and $beta_2$. $Beta_1$ receptors are present mainly in the heart and $beta_2$ are found in the lungs, blood vessels, and elsewhere in the body. Certain beta-blockers (such as atenolol, bisoprolol and metoprolol) are termed cardioselective and, because they act mostly on $beta_1$ receptors, are used principally to treat heart disease such as angina, hypertension, and cardiac *arrhythmia* (abnormal heartbeat). These drugs are sometimes given following a *myocardial infarction* (heart attack) in order to reduce the likelihood of further damage to the heart muscle.

Other types of beta-blocker, such as oxprenolol, propranolol, and timolol, may be given to prevent *migraine* attacks by acting on blood vessels in the head. They are also used to reduce the physical symptoms of *anxiety* and to control the symptoms of *thyrotoxicosis* (an overactive thyroid gland). Beta-blockers such as timolol are sometimes given in the form of eye-drops to treat *glaucoma*; they work by lowering the fluid pressure within the eyeball.

POSSIBLE ADVERSE EFFECTS
Beta-blocker drugs may reduce an individual's capacity for strenuous exercise. They may worsen the symptoms of *asthma*, *bronchitis*, or other forms of lung disease. They may also reduce the flow of blood to the limbs, causing cold hands and feet. In addition, sleep disturbance and depression can be side effects of beta-blockers. Anyone taking beta-blockers should not stop suddenly; a severe recurrence of previous symptoms and a significant rise in blood pressure may result. (See box, left.)

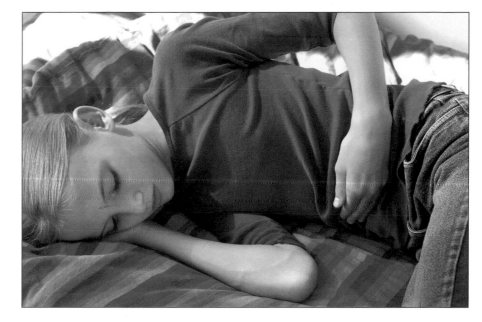

*Bezoar is a condition in which an indigestible ball of food and mucus, fibre, and/or hair forms in the stomach. The condition may cause abdominal pain.*

## Betahistine

A drug that is used in the treatment of the inner-ear disorder *Ménière's disease*. Betahistine reduces the frequency and severity of the characteristic attacks of nausea and vertigo.

## Beta interferon

A type of *interferon* (a protein produced naturally by body cells) sometimes used in the treatment of *multiple sclerosis*.

## Beta-lactam antibiotics

A group of antibiotic drugs that includes the penicillins and the cephalosporins. They work by altering chemical activity in bacteria, thereby killing them.

## Beta-lactamase

An enzyme, also known as lactamase, that inactivates antibiotic drugs such as penicillins. Bacteria that are able to produce this enzyme are therefore resistant to treatment with these kinds of antibiotic drugs.

## Betamethasone

A *corticosteroid drug* that is used in the treatment of inflammation. Corticosteroids work by blocking the production of natural substances that trigger inflammation, such as prostaglandins. Betamethasone is applied to the skin as a cream to treat contact *dermatitis* and *eczema*. The drug is also prescribed as a nasal spray to treat allergic *rhinitis* (hay fever) and is taken by mouth to treat some cases of *asthma* and *arthritis*.

Adverse effects are unlikely with short-term use. However, prolonged topical use of the drug can cause thinning of the skin and may aggravate any infection that has developed. Taken orally over a prolonged period or in high doses, betamethasone can cause adverse effects typical of other corticosteroid drugs.

## Bezoar

A ball of food and mucus, vegetable fibre, hair, or other indigestible material in the stomach. Trichobezoars, which are composed of hair, may form in the stomachs of children or emotionally disturbed adults who nibble at, or pull out and swallow, their hair.

Symptoms include loss of appetite, constipation, nausea and vomiting, and abdominal pain. If trichobezoars pass into the intestines, they may cause a blockage (see *intestine, obstruction of*). Bezoars can be removed by *endoscopy* (a procedure in which a flexible flexible tube is passed down the digestive tract) or by conventional surgery.

## Bicarbonate of soda

See *sodium bicarbonate*.

## Biceps muscle

The name that is given to any muscle that originates as two separate parts, which then fuse. The term biceps muscle is commonly used to refer to the biceps brachii muscle of the upper arm, which bends the arm at the elbow and rotates the forearm.

Another example of a biceps muscle is the biceps femoris muscle, which is located at the back of the thigh. this muscle bends the leg at the knee and extends the thigh.

**Using muscles**
*The biceps brachii muscle is evident here at the front of the upper arm; its opposing muscle, the triceps, is at the back of the arm. Both are involved in bending and straightening the arm.*

## Bicornuate uterus

The term that is used to describe an abnormally shaped uterus (womb) that divides into two halves in its upper part. Bicornuate literally means "having two horns".

## Bicuspid

A term meaning to have two cusps (curved, pointed structures). Bicuspid describes certain heart valves and is used as an alternative name for a premolar tooth (see *teeth*).

## Bifocal

A spectacle lens with two different focal lengths. Glasses that have bifocal lenses make corrections both for close and for distant vision. (See also *myopia*; *hypermetropia*.)

## Biguanides

Oral hypoglycaemic drugs (see *hypoglycaemics, oral*) used in the treatment of type 2 (non-insulin-dependent) *diabetes mellitus*. Metformin, which is the only available type of biguanide drug, reduces the production of glucose (sugar) in the liver and also increases the uptake of glucose by the body's cells. (See also *antidiabetic drugs*.)

## Bilateral

A term that means affecting both sides of the body, or affecting both organs if they are paired (for example, both ears are affected in bilateral deafness).

## Bile

A greenish-brown alkaline liquid that is secreted by the *liver*. Bile carries away waste products formed in the liver and also helps to break down fats in the small intestine for digestion.

The waste products in bile include the pigments *bilirubin* and biliverdin, which give bile its greenish brown colour; bile salts, which aid in the breakdown and absorption of fats; and *cholesterol*. Bile passes out of the liver through the *bile ducts* and is then concentrated and stored in the gall-bladder. After a meal, bile is expelled and enters the duodenum (the first section of the small intestine) via the common bile duct. Most of the bile salts are later reabsorbed into the bloodstream to be recycled by the liver into bile. Bile pigments are excreted in the faeces. (See also *biliary system*; *colestyramine*.)

## Bile duct

Any of the ducts through which *bile* is carried from the *liver* to the gall-bladder and then on to the duodenum (the first section of the small intestine).

The bile duct system forms a network of tubular canals. Canaliculi (small canals) surround the liver cells and collect the bile. The canaliculi join together to form ducts of increasing size. The ducts emerge from the liver as the two hepatic ducts, which join within or just outside the liver to form the common hepatic duct. The cystic duct branches off to the gallbladder; from this point the common hepatic duct becomes the common bile duct and leads into the duodenum. (See also *biliary system*.)

## Bile duct cancer

See *cholangiocarcinoma*.

## Bile duct obstruction

A blockage or constriction of a bile duct (see *biliary system*). Obstruction of a bile duct results in accumulation of bile in the liver (*cholestasis*) and jaundice (yellowing of the skin and the whites of the eyes) due to a buildup of

B

## THE BILIARY SYSTEM

Consisting of the bile ducts leading from the liver and gallbladder, the gallbladder itself, and associated structures, the biliary system drains waste products from the liver into the duodenum and aids the process of fat digestion through controlled release of fat-emulsifying agents that are contained in bile.

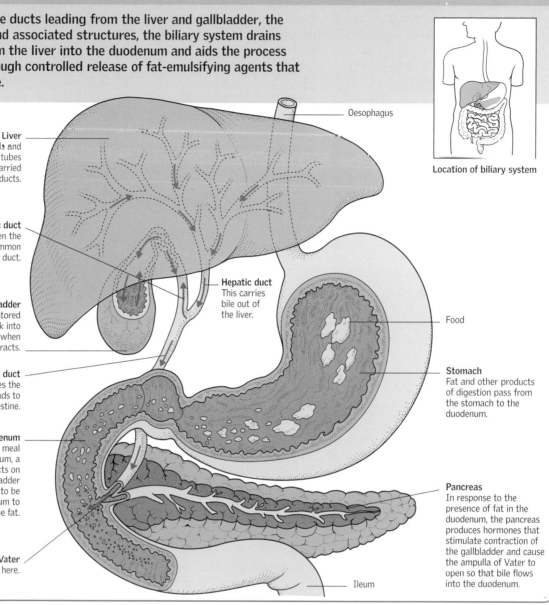

Location of biliary system

**Oesophagus**

**Liver**
Bile is secreted by liver cells and collected in a system of tubes (drainage channels). Bile is carried out of the liver via the hepatic ducts.

**Cystic duct**
This carries bile between the gallbladder and the common bile duct.

**Hepatic duct**
This carries bile out of the liver.

**Gallbladder**
Bile is concentrated and stored here and is released back into the common bile duct when this organ contracts.

**Food**

**Common bile duct**
The hepatic duct becomes the common bile duct, which leads to the intestine.

**Stomach**
Fat and other products of digestion pass from the stomach to the duodenum.

**Duodenum**
When fat from a recent meal arrives in the duodenum, a hormone is released that acts on the gallbladder. The gallbladder contracts, causing bile to be passed into the duodenum to emulsify the fat.

**Pancreas**
In response to the presence of fat in the duodenum, the pancreas produces hormones that stimulate contraction of the gallbladder and cause the ampulla of Vater to open so that bile flows into the duodenum.

**Ampulla of Vater**
Bile enters the duodenum here.

**Ileum**

*bilirubin* (bile pigment) in the blood. Prolonged obstruction of the bile duct can lead to secondary biliary cirrhosis, a serious form of liver disease.

## CAUSES

The most common cause of bile duct obstruction is *gallstones*, which develop when there is a disturbance in the chemical composition of bile. Other causes include a tumour affecting the pancreas (see *pancreas, cancer of*) and cancer that has spread from elsewhere in the body. *Cholangiocarcinoma* (cancer of the bile ducts) is a rare cause of a blockage. Bile duct obstruction is known to be a rare side effect of certain drugs. It may also be caused by *cholangitis* (inflammation of the bile ducts), trauma (such as injury during surgery), and, rarely, by *flukes* or worms.

## SYMPTOMS

Bile duct obstruction causes "obstructive" jaundice, which is characterized by pale-coloured faeces, dark urine, and a yellow skin colour. There may also be itching. Other symptoms of bile-duct obstruction depend on the cause of the blockage; for example, there may be abdominal pain (with gallstones) or weight loss (with cancer).

## TREATMENT

Treatment depends on the cause, but surgery is sometimes necessary. Gallstones may be removed by means of *ERCP* (an X-ray procedure that uses a viewing tube called an endoscope with instruments attached to it).

# Bilharzia

Another name for the tropical parasitic disease *schistosomiasis*.

# Biliary atresia

A rare *congenital* disorder in which some or all of the *bile ducts* fail to develop or develop abnormally. As a result, bile is unable to drain from the liver (see *cholestasis*). Unless the atresia can be treated, secondary *biliary cirrhosis* (a serious liver disorder) will develop and may prove fatal. Symptoms include *jaundice*, usually beginning a week after birth, and the passing of dark urine and pale faeces. Treatment is by surgery to bypass the ducts. If this fails, or if the jaundice recurs, a *liver transplant* is required.

# Biliary cirrhosis

An uncommon form of liver *cirrhosis* that results from problems with the bile ducts. There are two types of biliary cirrhosis. One is an *autoimmune disorder* and is known as primary biliary cirrhosis. Secondary biliary cirrhosis occurs as a result of a long-standing blockage. In both types of the condition, liver function is impaired due to *cholestasis* (accumulation of bile in the liver).

Primary biliary cirrhosis principally affects middle-aged women and seems to be linked with a malfunction of the *immune system*. In this disorder, the bile ducts within the liver become inflamed and are destroyed. Symptoms of the condition include itching, *jaundice* (a yellowish discoloration of the skin and the whites of the eyes), an enlarged liver, and sometimes abdominal pain, fatty diarrhoea, and *xanthomatosis* (deposits of fatty material under the skin). *Osteoporosis* may also develop.

Symptoms of liver cirrhosis and *liver failure* may occur after a few years. Drugs can be used to minimize complications and to relieve symptoms such as itching, but a *liver transplant* is the only cure.

Secondary biliary cirrhosis results from prolonged *bile duct obstruction* or *biliary atresia* (abnormal bile ducts). Symptoms and signs of this condition include abdominal pain and tenderness, liver enlargement, fevers and chills, and sometimes blood abnormalities. Treatment for secondary biliary cirrhosis is the same as for bile duct obstruction.

# Biliary colic

A severe pain in the upper right quadrant of the abdomen that is usually caused by the gallbladder's attempts to expel *gallstones* or by the movement of a stone in the *bile ducts*. The pain may be felt in the right shoulder (see *referred pain*) or may penetrate to the centre of the back. Episodes of biliary colic often last for several hours and may recur, particularly after meals.

Injections of an *analgesic drug* and *antispasmodic drug* may be given to relieve the colic. Tests such as *cholecystography* or *ultrasound scanning* can confirm the presence of gallstones, in which case *cholecystectomy* (surgical removal of the gallbladder) may be performed.

# Biliary system

The organs and ducts in which *bile* is formed, concentrated, and carried from the *liver* to the duodenum (the first part of the small intestine). Bile is secreted by liver cells and collected by a network of *bile ducts* that carry the bile out of the liver via the hepatic duct. The cystic duct branches off the hepatic duct and leads to the bladder, where the bile is concentrated and stored. Beyond this junction, the hepatic duct becomes the common bile duct, which opens into the

duodenum at a controlled orifice known as the ampulla of Vater. The presence of fat in the duodenum following a meal prompts the secretion of a hormone that opens the ampulla of Vater. This causes contraction of the gallbladder, which squeezes stored bile into the duodenum.

The main disorders affecting the biliary system are *gallstones*, congenital *biliary atresia* and *bile duct obstruction*. (See box on previous page; see also *gallbladder, disorders of*.)

# Biliousness

A condition in which bile is brought up to the mouth from the stomach. Biliousness is also used as a non-medical term for nausea and vomiting.

# Bilirubin

The main pigment in *bile*. Bilirubin is produced by the breakdown of *haemoglobin*, the pigment in red blood cells. Very high levels of bilirubin cause the yellow pigmentation of *jaundice*. Products formed from the breakdown of bilirubin make faeces brown.

# Billings' method

Also known as the mucus inspection method, the Billings' method is a technique in which a woman notes changes in the characteristics of mucus produced by her cervix. The technique is employed to predict ovulation for the purposes of contraception or family planning.

# Billroth's operation

A type of partial *gastrectomy* in which the lower part of the stomach is surgically removed. Previously used in the treatment of *peptic ulcers*, the operation is now rarely performed due to the introduction of newer, less invasive treatment, often using antibiotic drugs.

## BIOENERGETICS

Bioenergetics is a body-oriented form of psychotherapy developed in the US in the 1960s by Dr. Alexander Lowen. An individual's history of dealing with stress or trauma is thought to be "programmed" into the muscles, and practitioners believe that posture and physical tension provide clues to mental attitudes and psychological problems. Bioenergetics exaggerates then releases tension linked with buried memories, enabling past traumas to be explored. Known as Bioenergetic Analysis in North America, where most practitioners are based, bioenergetics is also practised in Europe and in New Zealand.

### History

The term "bioenergetics" was first coined by Dr. Alexander Lowen, a US psychotherapist practising in the 1960s. He was a student of Wilhelm Reich, who was a follower of Freud. Reich believed that the body, mind, and emotions are deeply interrelated. To develop bioenergetics, Dr. Lowen adapted some of Reich's ideas, including his theory of "body-armouring" (adopting defensive postures because of past events). Someone hurt as a child, for example, might hold herself as if warding off blows. Following Freud's practice of encouraging people to relive repressed traumas, Dr. Lowen devised exercises from sources such as t'ai chi ch'uan and Pilates.

### Consulting a practitioner

After an initial one-to-one assessment, the practitioner may recommend individual therapy sessions, joining a group, or a combination of the two approaches. A session may last roughly 50 minutes and comfortable clothing should be worn.

### Releasing emotions

*Physical tension is released in exercises like wringing a towel, or hitting a bed with a bat or racquet, which allow the patient to vent her emotions. Such confrontational work can release anger, frustration, or grief.*

Workshops usually contain between 12 and 20 people, and may begin with warm-up movements before a sharing of experiences. Exercises focus on tense areas, such as a "frozen" chest, "locked" pelvis, and tension in the jaw. Attention is paid to "grounding" – the way you stand and balance – as practitioners believe that if you are in firm touch with the ground, you will also be in touch with your body and emotions. Key "stress positions", like lying backwards over a stool, are often used to build up and unlock emotional energy. Repressed memories may surface during the course of these exercises, and there may be outpourings of emotion.

### Grounding

*The patient stands and stretches up, supported by the practitioner. She focuses on feeling the ground beneath her, and on her body and emotions.*

### Evidence and research

A number of papers on bioenergetic theories and practice have been published in psychotherapeutic journals, but most evidence is anecdotal: six sessions can be life-changing for some people, while others continue for years.

The patient pulls and wrings a rolled towel to release emotion or aggression

The practitioner encourages the patient to express her feelings

### Medical opinion

If body and mind are as closely linked as practitioners suggest, then the theory of bioenergetics is plausible. Any doctor would appreciate that strong feelings may manifest physically – we talk of "tension" headaches, "irritable" bowel and "nervous" stomachs. But the defences that cause feelings to be expressed through the body, rather than directly, are very important, and doctors are concerned that they should be dismantled only at a pace that the patient can handle.

B

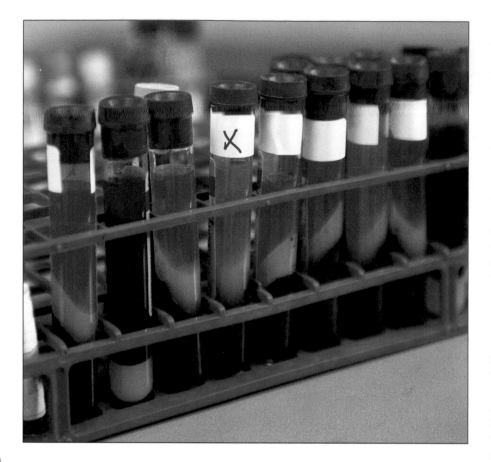

**Biochemistry** *teaches us about the chemical changes going on in cells from measurements of the minerals, gases, enzymes, hormones, and proteins in blood, urine, and other body fluids.*

## Binge–purge syndrome

An alternative term for the eating disorder *bulimia*.

## Bioavailability

The proportion of a drug that reaches the target organs and tissues, usually expressed as a percentage of the dose administered. Intravenous administration of a drug results in 100 per cent bioavailability because the drug is injected directly into the bloodstream. Drugs taken orally have a much lower bioavailability. Preparations that have equal bioavailabilities are described as bioequivalent. (See also *drug*.)

## Biochemistry

A science that studies the chemistry of living organisms, including human beings. The human body is made up of millions of cells that require nutrients and energy, and which grow, multiply, and die. The chemical processes that are involved in providing these cells with energy, eliminating their wastes, repairing damage, promoting cell growth, and causing both normal and abnormal cell division are all studied by biochemists, who are the specialists in the field.

Life is maintained by a huge number of chemical reactions that are carried out inside cells. These reactions link together in a complex way and together make up the *metabolism* of the body. The reactions that produce energy and break down food and body structures are termed catabolism; those that build up body structures and store food are termed anabolism. Overall regulation of these chemical processes is a principal function of *hormones* which are secreted into the bloodstream by the *endocrine glands*; regulation of individual reactions is carried out by *enzymes* (substances that promote biochemical reactions).

Certain vital chemical processes take place in every single cell in the body. Other, more specific, chemical processes are confined to specialized cells that make up the tissues of particular organs. For example, liver cells store and chemically modify the digestion products of food; kidney cells help to control the amounts of various substances (such as certain minerals) in the blood, as well as regulating the total amount of fluid in the body.

A constant interchange of substances occurs between the cell fluids and the blood and urine. Biochemists can learn a great deal about the chemical changes occurring inside the body's cells by regularly taking, and comparing, precise measurements of the various minerals, gases, enzymes, hormones, and proteins in the different fluids of the body.

Such biochemical tests may be used to make, or to confirm, a diagnosis, as well as to screen for a particular disease and to monitor its progress. The most commonly used biochemical tests are performed on *blood*; such tests include *liver function tests* and *kidney function tests*. Biochemical tests can also be performed on urine (see urinalysis) as well as on all other body fluids.

## Bioenergetics

See box on previous page.

## Bioengineering

See *biomechanical engineering*.

## Biofeedback

See box opposite.

# BIOFEEDBACK

In the 1960s, US scientists began training people to control heart-rate and other unconscious biological functions by using electronic "biofeedback" instruments that monitor subtle physical responses. Electrodes or probes are used to attach patients to the biofeedback device, and signals, such as electronic beeps, flashes, or needles on a dial, "feed back" information about changes in the body. By responding to these signals, patients can learn to self-regulate body functions. The technique may help to treat stress-related conditions, including certains types of hypertension (high blood pressure), anxiety, and migraine.

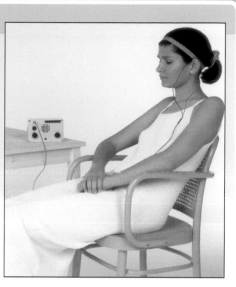

*An electroencephalograph (EEG) uses electrodes attached to the scalp to record the complex series of electrical charges produced by brain-wave activity.*

### History

In the early 1930s, scientists in the US and UK developed electronic devices to detect minute physical responses. At first, publicity focused on obtaining electrical signals from the brain, but the work of US scientists in the 1960s confirmed the therapeutic value of biofeedback.

Drs. Elmer and Alyce Green of the Menninger Foundation, Kansas, used the method to study states of mind during yoga meditation, and by the 1980s stress-management courses using biofeedback had been introduced in some US primary schools. Advances in computer technology are prompting further research.

### Consulting a practitioner

The practitioner will show you how to use the biofeedback device, of which there are several types: a skin temperature (ST) gauge registers heat changes in the skin; a galvanic skin response (GSR) sensor measures the skin's electrical conductivity by the amount of sweat produced under stress; electromyographs (EMGs) use auditory or visual signals to indicate muscle tension; electroencephalographs (EEGs) show brain-wave activity; and electro-cardiographs (ECGs) monitor heart-rate.

After some experience with the technique, the person starts to become aware of how he or she is feeling whenever there is a change of signal. By using relaxation techniques, such as

breathing and muscle relaxation, the person learns to change the signals by conscious control of the function. A state of relaxation is indicated by warm skin, low sweat-gland activity, high levels of alpha waves from the brain, and a slow, even heart-rate. Biofeedback takes practice; at least six half-hour sessions may be needed.

### Evidence and research

An extensive body of clinical researchs support the claims of biofeedback. A 1996 study in the US showed that using the technique to relax shoulder muscles could ease tension headaches. In 1992, a US study showed that muscular pain in the lower back responded to biofeedback, and a US government report in 1992 found that patients could control incontinence with the technique. It is being used at Yale University to control heart-rate and blood pressure and some US doctors are using it to treat epilepsy.

### Medical opinion

In the past, few doctors would have believed that people could learn to influence their blood pressure or brain-waves. Today, the evidence is conclusive and biofeedback's entry into the medical mainstream seems inevitable, although some doctors continue to question its reliability as a form of treatment.

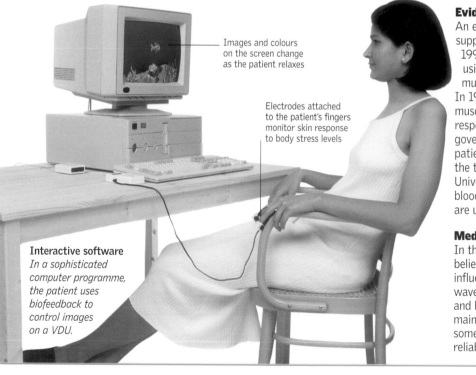

Images and colours on the screen change as the patient relaxes

Electrodes attached to the patient's fingers monitor skin response to body stress levels

**Interactive software**
*In a sophisticated computer programme, the patient uses biofeedback to control images on a VDU.*

B

# Picture Credits

**Front and back cover images © Dorling Kindersley Ltd.**

**Spine image: AKG-Images/Cameraphoto.**